...th Recovery

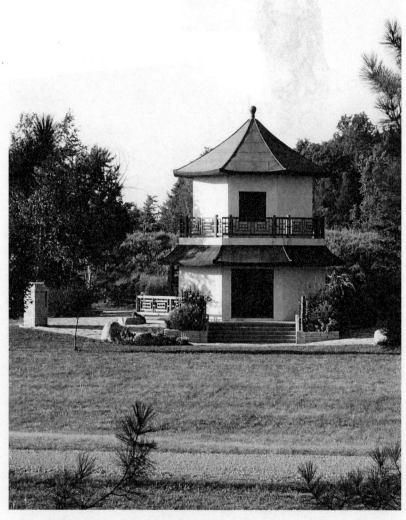

Columbarium housing the ashes of Master Moy and others
(Thanks to Andy Ferenc for the location for taking the photo)

Health Recovery
The *Taoist Tai Chi*™ Way

ROD GIBLETT

SHEPHEARD-WALWYN (PUBLISHERS) LTD

First published in 2008 by
Shepheard-Walwyn (Publishers) Ltd
15 Alder Road
London SW14 8ER

British Library Cataloguing in Publication Data
A catalogue record of this book
is available from the British Library

ISBN-13: 978-0-85683-259-8

Taoist Tai Chi™ and Taoist Tai Chi Society™ are trademarks of
Certmark Holdings Co. Ltd. used under licence by the
International Taoist Tai Chi Society and its member organisations,
in relation to the instruction of various internal arts of health
transmitted by Moy Lin-shin.

Typeset by Heavens and Earth Art,
Alderton, Suffolk
Printed and bound through
s|s| media limited, Wallington, Surrey

Dedicated to the Memory of
Master Moy Lin-Shin (1931-1998)

Founder of the International Taoist Tai Chi Society
and the Gei Pang Lok Hup Academy
Co-Founder of the Fung Loy Kok Institute of Taoism

DISCLAIMER

The author, Rod Giblett, is a member of the Taoist Tai Chi Society of Australia. As a personal endeavour he has conducted the research for, and the writing of, this book. The views expressed herein are personal to him or the persons he has interviewed, and they remain his sole responsibility. They do not necessarily represent the views of the Taoist Tai Chi Society of Australia, the Taoist Tai Chi Society of Canada, the International Taoist Tai Chi Society or any other of their respective members (collectively, the "Society"). The Society accepts no responsibility for the views expressed by the author or the persons he has interviewed. The work of the reference group established by the Society in order to review the process and comment on drafts, and the rights of access granted to the author by the Society for the purposes of his work, do not constitute in anyway an implicit or explicit support for such views. The author is also solely responsible for the accuracy of the statements attributed to interviewees and conveyed in this book. The practice of the exercises and techniques alluded to in this book, like any form of physical training, entails risks of physical injury and such risks depend on one's physical and mental condition and the degree of care that is applied in training. The Society accepts no liability for any damages or injuries incurred as a result of attempting to practice such exercises and techniques. To minimize such risks, the reader wishing to engage in such practice is invited to do so under the supervision of a qualified instructor.

CONTENTS

Acknowledgments

I am grateful to Edith Cowan University for granting me paid study leave for a year and financial support for travel to Canada and the US in order to undertake research for, and to complete the bulk of the writing of, this book. I am especially grateful to Professor Robyn Quin, the Executive Dean of the Faculty of Communications and Creative Industries, for extending my Study Leave so that I was able to complete the writing of two drafts of the book during this period.

The planning for, and carrying out of, this project through the research, writing, editing and publication phases was guided and overseen by a reference group from the International Taoist Tai Chi Society comprising: Dr Peter Cook, then President (now Executive Director) of the Taoist Tai Chi Society of Australia and Chair of the International Taoist Tai Chi Society Publications Committee; Heath Greville, Director of the International Taoist Tai Chi Society (and my first teacher of Taoist Tai Chi™* taijiquan and Lok Hup Ba Fa); Sandy Morrison, President of the Taoist Tai Chi Society of New Zealand; Jennifer Lefroy, then President of the Taoist Tai Chi Society of Western Australia; Kelly Ekman, Administrator of the International Taoist Tai Chi Society Health Recovery Centre in Canada; and Dr Bruce McFarlane, Medical Director of the Centre.

I am grateful to the reference group for their input and advice, especially in the early stages when it was doubtful that we would be able to design a project that was mutually acceptable and in the later stages for their helpful comments and suggestions on the written drafts. All failures to follow their suggestions regarding style and content are entirely my own responsibility. All blame for the results of these failings lies with me.

I am also very grateful to the people I interviewed for giving generously of their time and energy to talk to me. Peter Turner was especially helpful in transcribing some of the interview with him and correcting and clarifying some points in the rest that I had transcribed, and in the rest of the book. I am grateful to him and to Helen Gaunt, James Matthews and Ian Shaw for providing their testimonials and for giving permission for their republication. Sean Dennison and Philippe Gagnon were appointed as readers by the board of the International Taoist Tai Chi Society. I am grateful to Sean for reading and making amendments and corrections to the penultimate draft, to Philippe for the disclaimer and to Sean for suggesting that I interview Judy Millen and Dee Steverson, both key 'informants.' I am also grateful for the companionship, support, advice, suggestions and comments of Sandra Giblett through all the stages of this project. Finally, I gratefully acknowledge Mr Moy as the source and master of Taoist Tai Chi™ taijiquan, as the teacher of other Taoist arts of health and as the founder of the International Taoist Tai Chi Society and other organizations devoted to other Taoist arts (hence the dedication of this book to his memory).

ONE

Introduction

Beginnings

*T*HE ANCIENT Chinese art of Tai Chi, or *taijiquan*, is now widely recognised in Western, industrialised countries and some of its benefits are readily acknowledged. The slow, graceful movements of *taijiquan* are so well-known that they are occasionally used in television advertisements often just to signify relaxation or a healthy life-style. *Taijiquan* is visually appealing and people who watch it often remark that it looks relaxing. More importantly, the people who do it often say that it feels relaxing, and is relaxing too. Yet these practitioners often have a lot more to say about its effects on them. This book gathers together the stories of some people who practise *Taoist Tai Chi*™ *taijiquan* and other *Taoist Tai Chi*™ internal arts of health, and who talk about their benefits for them.

Many people will have heard that *taijiquan* is good for relieving arthritis, or for improving balance, or reducing high blood pressure, or preventing osteoporosis, or helping with a range of other conditions. People who practise the *Taoist Tai Chi*™ internal arts of health sometimes have these, or other, incurable or terminal, conditions such as Lou Gehrig's syndrome, Multiple Sclerosis, Cerebral Palsy, Alzheimer's, or have had cancer or a stroke. This book presents the stories of some people who have some of these conditions. Other people start practising these arts because they are unfit and want to get fit; overweight and want to lose weight; and even because they are healthy and want to stay healthy, especially as they get older.

There are no miraculous cures to be had through the practice of these arts, but there can be, and are, remarkable transformational experiences and big improvements in functionality, even with the simple functions of everyday life, which many of us take for granted, such as walking and even standing. There are improvements in balance, strength and flexibility, and in a general sense of wellbeing, giving improved quality and increased length of life. Examples of this wide range of experience were recorded and are presented in this book.

Taijiquan is taught in a number of 'styles' or traditions. *Taoist Tai Chi™ taijiquan* is taught by the International Taoist Tai Chi Society ('the Society'). It emphasises the health-restoring and -maintaining aspects of *taijiquan* and other Taoist arts of health and well-being. Health-improvement is one of the core aims of the Society. Health, however, is not defined in this book (nor by the Society, I would suggest) in narrow, physical terms, but in broad, holistic terms that include physical, mental, spiritual, emotional, and even environmental health. These arts focus on the physical as the initial means to recover health in the other areas as well. Change the body to change the mind and spirit is a motto of the tradition of Taoism from which these arts and the Society and its teachings come.

Taoist Tai Chi™ taijiquan has a number of specific and demonstrable benefits. It is described in an old brochure published by the Taoist Tai Chi Society of Australia as:

a gentle art of health for people of all ages and health conditions. The slow, graceful movements of Taoist Tai Chi increase strength and flexibility and improve balance and circulation. The Taoist style of Tai Chi emphasises stretching and turning in each of the movements in order to gain these and other benefits more effectively.

The brochure goes on to relate that:

Regular practice of Taoist Tai Chi can bring a wide range of health benefits to the muscular, skeletal and circulatory systems. The flowing movements of Taoist Tai Chi serve as a moving meditation that reduces stress and provides a way to cultivate body and mind. Specific health benefits include:

- toning of muscles, tendons and other soft tissues;
- rotation of the joints through a full range of motion;
- stretching and alignment of the spine to make it strong and supple;
- gentle massage of the internal organs to improve their functioning.

This book documents these and other benefits anecdotally and auto-biographically.

Taoist Tai Chi™ *taijiquan* and other internal arts of health were developed by Master Moy Lin-Shin (1931-1998) and brought to the West in 1970 when he initially founded the Taoist Tai Chi Society of Canada and later the International Taoist Tai Chi Society. Since then the Society has grown to be the largest non-profit, volunteer *taijiquan* organization in the world. These arts are practised in over 25 countries and 500 locations around the world, mainly in Europe, North America and Australia.

The people who tell their stories in this book come from these three continents. They were asked three questions in order to focus and direct the conversation: Why did you start learning *Taoist Tai Chi*™ *taijiquan*? Why do you continue practising it? What effect has practising it had on you? Answering these questions often involved the storytellers talking about the context in which these reasons and effects occur, and how that context contributes to producing the effects and reinforcing the reasons for continuing with the practice of this art. This context includes the experience of learning this art and being a part of the International Taoist Tai Chi Society. Practising this art is not an isolated, individual experience, but takes place in the context of the community of the Society. For this reason the storytellers usually talk about their experience of being a member of the Society, or of participating in a Health Recovery Program at a Society Centre. They also talk about how either or both being a member and participant contribute to improving their health and well-being. The reasons for continuing to practise this art and experiencing its effects are related to this context. These effects are largely expressed as benefits in physical health, and mental and spiritual well-being. The desire to gain those benefits is often the reason for taking up this art in the first place.

The Society is thus the context in which the benefits of practising this art are nurtured. As Master Moy founded the Society, his teaching and vision are the source of those benefits, including the health benefits. Tracing the lineage of this art and the Society back to its source in Master Moy is not only the respectful thing to do, but also establishes the legitimacy and power of the practice and its health benefits. It is an important aspect of this art, and of the ongoing teaching of it, that an accomplished master taught it initially and did so for many years. The students of Master Moy hold him in great respect.

Master Moy, however, was not your stereotype of the guru who dressed flashily, drove a big car and lived a lavish lifestyle. He usually wore a Society tee-shirt and a track-suit with the Society logo on it. He never took a salary and he lived a very simple life. He also did not adopt the master position in which he was the all-seeing, all-knowing master on to whom the student transferred their desires and fears. Who and what he was will be discussed later, especially in the chapter devoted to him. Some of the storytellers in this book talk about their experience of meeting Master Moy and what their impressions of him were. They often go on to talk about specific 'corrections' to their *taijiquan* that he made, or other directions that he had given to them, both of which contributed to their recovering, or maintaining, their health, and to their life story. Some other storytellers who did not meet him talk about their impressions of him too.

Besides founding the Society and being the source of *Taoist Tai Chi™ taijiquan* and other arts of health and well-being, Master Moy also taught chanting and meditation. The Society offers instruction and practice in both at some locations as part of the Taoist lineage and heritage. These health-improving practices are complementary with the other arts and integral to the activities of the Society, to the process of health recovery and to stories about it. Some people tell their stories about chanting and meditation, and about the effects either, or both, have had on them. Generally the people who say they have received the most benefit (physically and spiritually) from membership of, and/or participation in the activities of, the Society are those who practise chanting and meditation as well as *Taoist Tai Chi™ taijiquan* and other arts.

The storytellers are a small, selective (non-random) sample of practitioners from various types of classes, programs and workshops. Their stories explore the motivation for practising these arts. In particular, the stories explore the reasons why these people chose these arts, their experience of practising them and their perception of the contribution that they have made to their lives. They also make observations about the teaching and learning of these arts and about the nature and functioning of classes and programs at Society sites. From these stories common themes are identified and discussed, and conclusions drawn about these arts and the Society.

This book not only presents these individual stories, but also tries to convey the experience of participating in the activities of the Society and the benefits gained from practising these arts, especially as a participant at a Health Recovery Program conducted by the Society. This is the only program of instruction in these arts offered to non-members. Anyone can come along and try them for themselves. These arts are usually accessible only to those who become members of the Society. Classes are not offered on a fee-for-service basis, but on the basis of membership dues. The philosophy behind the Society is that it is not a *taijiquan* club, but a social, spiritual and community organization that is, and does, a lot more than *taijiquan*. These arts are not a commodity the consumer can buy. Members pay dues to belong to the Society and membership entitles them to instruction and participation in a class.

Background

The background to the research for this book was that I had been investigating the Taoist body, Taoist ecology and illness narratives, or pathographies. These are personal accounts of illness, written usually by the person with the illness (auto-pathography). They usually recount an experience with illness that starts with a diagnosis, searching for, and possibly finding, a cure, undergoing surgery or other treatment, and ends with living with the illness, or in death. They are elaborated, written and published narratives. They are published in either books or magazines. Journalists, novelists and sociologists largely write those published in book-form about themselves. They have the writing expertise and experience, and access to publishers, needed to produce books. Of course, there are exceptions to this rule with the odd champion cyclist thrown in such as Lance Armstrong, but in such cases celebrity status greases the wheels of publication. Illness narratives published in magazines are written either by journalists about celebrities, or by non-celebrities about themselves with some editorial or journalistic assistance. They are all amazing and inspiring stories of bravery and heroism in the face of incredible odds, sometimes with remarkable results.

From my experience of practising the *Taoist Tai Chi*™ internal arts of health and of being an instructor *Taoist Tai Chi*™ taijiquan for more than 20 years, I knew that there were other stories being told by practitioners of recovered and maintained health, or improved quality and increased length of life. Unlike the illness narrative where the narrator often has an operable or potentially curable condition such as cancer, many of the tellers of what could be called 'health recovery stories' have inoperable or incurable conditions such as MS or ALS. Cancer lends itself to the typical trajectory of the illness narrative wherein the narrator descends into the murky underworld of the hospital and clinic to emerge triumphant or vanquished in the end, with or without the assistance of medical and nursing helpers.

By contrast, the health recovery story is a story without the same peaks and troughs, beginnings and endings. It is a story of ups and downs, occasional breakthroughs and setbacks in trying to improve health, always with the assistance and help of instructors and others in the same boat. Health recovery stories are unelaborated, oral and largely unpublished accounts told by people from a range of backgrounds with different expertise and experience. Some of these stories of health recovery or improvement have been told in 'testimonials' published in newsletters by the Society or have circulated in oral form amongst members and practitioners. They have not been told to the wider public. This book tells some of those health recovery stories more widely. It also includes some testimonials.

However, this book does not just present individual health recovery stories in isolation. The chapters are not organized around individual people, though they are divided into sections for each informant. These sections foreground a theme mentioned by these people. The chapters are organised around common topics and concerns that emerged from listening to, transcribing, reading, and rereading, the stories. These are more to do with Taoism and the International Taoist Tai Chi Society than just with *Taoist Tai Chi*™ *taijiquan*. This book presents Taoism as a biospiritual practice, or cultivation, involving a holistic transformation of mind, body and spirit. Similarly, body, mind and spirit are nurtured within and by the culture and community of the International Taoist Tai Chi Society. Yet the benefits of this practice are not only experienced by those who call themselves 'Taoists' but are readily available to all who practise this *taijiquan* and are members of the Society or participate in its programs. Health recovery stories are primarily stories about Taoism and the International Taoist Tai Chi Society, and not just about *taijiquan*. The book, as conveyed in its title and sub-title, focuses on this and others arts as a way to gain access to, and stimulate interest in, and even inspire participation in, Taoism and the Society.

The Society is largely an oral culture where its activities take place in a face-to-face situation, including learning this art. In fact, it is recommended that everyone learns in a class, and not from a book or video. It is difficult, if not impossible, to learn from a book or video, though the Society has both available as they have a useful function to provide aids to memory about moves, and the sequence of moves, taught in a class. This present book, by contrast, tries to give a sense of the oral culture of the Society by presenting stories about it. These stories are excerpted from transcriptions of interviews, an oral genre. Of course, this book is a written account, too, like illness narratives. It is thus a pale imitation of actually talking to the people who told their stories initially face-to-face. Hopefully, though, it tells their stories adequately and gives a sense of their experience, and of the oral culture of the Society. A number of men and women, of different ages, from a variety of backgrounds, of various nationalities, in good or poor health (or somewhere between them) tell their stories. These stories show that the practice of the *Taoist Tai Chi*™ internal arts of health is not just for the old or young, mobile or immobile, sick or ill, fit or unfit. It is for everybody.

What other activity or club has members that range in age from 9 to 90, from those in the pink of health to those on death's door, from those who cannot feed themselves, stand up or walk unaided to those who do rolls, splits and headstands? And all this is done in a friendly, non-competitive and supportive environment.

Setting

The rolling hills of rural Ontario in Canada are the perfect location for the International Health Recovery Centre of the International Taoist Tai Chi Society. It is located in the Mono area near Orangeville, about a 35-40 minute drive north-west of Toronto. The peaceful atmosphere of the Centre and its grounds provide an ideal, and idyllic, retreat and refuge for people to focus and work on regaining and improving their health. The property is about 106 acres in size. It includes a secluded wood through which the Bruce Trail wends on its way from Niagara Falls to the tip of Bruce Peninsula.

I visited this Centre and stayed there for 6 weeks from July to September in 2003 when I was on Study Leave from Edith Cowan University in Perth, Western Australia. I also made a brief visit to the Taoist Tai Chi Society of the USA Centre in Tallahassee, Florida. The Orangeville Centre in Canada is unique and its work is invaluable (and all royalties from the sale of this book go to help support it). It provides rich opportunities for research into the *Taoist Tai Chi*™ internal arts of health not available elsewhere in the world as nothing like this Centre exists anywhere else. This book presents to outsiders for the first time insiders' stories about the Centre and the Society.

I visited the centre at Orangeville much like an anthropologist visits a remote tribe, studies their practices, rituals and life-ways, and then brings home the booty in the form of an ethnographic study comprising knowledge of that other culture. It is as if there is this strange tribe scattered around the world whose members practise some aspects of the ancient Chinese arts of healing. Generally members of the tribe have jobs and families, but occasionally some of them come to their Centre in Canada to work together intensively on their own *taijiquan*, to improve their health, and to teach and help others. I wanted to study the life and activities of this Centre and concentrate on the community and culture of the *Taoist Tai Chi*™ internal arts of health and of the Society, and only focus on individuals as the bearers of knowledge and as informants about both. The aim was not to showcase or privilege the experience of those individuals, but to use it as a means of presenting the culture and community of these arts and the Society as the context for health recovery and stories about it.

Of course, in the case of this ethnographic study, as a member of the Taoist Tai Chi Society of Australia and an instructor of *Taoist Tai Chi*™ *taijiquan* myself, I belong in some sense to the same (modern, Western) culture and (*Taoist Tai Chi*™) 'tribe.' Yet there are cultural differences between the various classes outlined above and between Canada and the US to which I travelled and Australia from where I came. I acknowledge and respect these differences and reflected critically on the process of the research, including in both recording observations and conducting interviews. As a member of the same 'tribe' (albeit in a remote location in Australia) I was not a dispassionate observer, but rather a participant observer conducting fieldwork in a semi-familiar place. It was familiar in the sense that the people practised this art like me; unfamiliar in the sense that they were practising it in Ontario and Florida in two countries (and indeed in a hemisphere) that I had not visited before. In technical terms, I was doing ethnography from within (if that is possible).

My function as ethnographer was to engage in dialogue with the interviewees and to allow them to tell their own stories. My role as writer has been to make observations, draw conclusions, avoid editorialising and generally let the storytellers speak directly to the reader without interruption. My position as author is not that of an objective reporter, but of an engaged advocate. I am too implicated and involved as an instructor of this *taijiquan* and office bearer of the Society, and have been for too long, to try to, or to pretend to, stand outside it and observe it from that point of view. This book is for outsiders with insiders' stories by an insider. For those who are interested, I reflect more on these aspects, and in more academic terms, in the final chapter.

Being a participant-observer was certainly the case during the first week I was at the Orangeville Centre. I arrived just before a five-day Health Recovery Program commenced. The Administrator of the Centre, Kelly Ekman and the Medical Director, Dr Bruce McFarlane, asked me to be a Participant for this week so that I could become familiar with a Health Recovery program. I attended two subsequent Health Recovery weeks, the next one as an Assistant and the final one as the researcher (and amateur photographer) for this book. Through this process I was able to learn about the operations of the Centre and the activities of a Health Recovery Program from the point of view of both a Participant and an Assistant. I was also able to make contact and develop trust with potential storytellers. I also kept a journal in which I made observations about the life, activities and people of the Centre, including some of the storytellers. Some of these observations are presented in the final chapter.

How did I choose the storytellers? Or how did they choose to become involved? The 'sample' selected is not random, though it is rather arbitrary. I wanted to interview a broad range of people on the continuums of age, health and mobility as I have indicated. There was a touch of serendipity to it. Some people who told me their stories I had met only 5 minutes before. Others had become friends over several weeks, and occasionally months, of practising the *Taoist Tai Chi*™ internal arts of health together, eating meals together, washing dishes together and enjoying conversation. The Centre at Orangeville is like that. People live together, work together, practise *taijiquan* and other arts together and share the common tasks of everyday life together. And have a lot of fun and laugh a lot doing them. Generally the storytellers were interested in the project and wanted to help out. People who practise these arts are like that. Sometimes I had heard that they had an interesting or remarkable story to tell that others should hear. At other times I didn't know much about them at all. Our paths crossed and we stopped for a chat that was recorded and later transcribed, some bits of which made their way into this book.

This book is a kind of photo album of snapshots showing people in certain places at particular times talking about their experience of practising the *Taoist Tai Chi*™ internal arts of health and being members of the Society or participants in its activities. It does not pretend to be representative of all the people, and their experiences, who practise these arts. Yet these stories have validity in their own right, though it is not possible to extrapolate from this small sample of informants and to generalise from them about these arts, the Society and its effects on people. The book aims to give a flavour of the range of what happens in the Society. If you go to these places and talk to these people, they may tell you something slightly different on any given day. If you go to these places and talk to different people, they may tell you something slightly different. If you go to different places and talk to different people, they will tell you something slightly different too. Every person's experience of practising these arts of health is different and unique. Yet there are some commonalities and some surprising similarities between what practitioners say about them, and what members of the Society say about them. Those commonalities and similarities will become apparent in more detail later.

It may be valuable at this point to indicate a common theme in order to set the scene for what follows. One of the major, common characteristics that the storytellers repeatedly talked about is the social solidarity and support that the International Taoist Tai Chi Society provides to them and other members. The Society is a kind of second family and second home for many people that adds to, or replaces, their first family and home, which could be unsatisfactory or unsupportive or no longer available or in existence. This sense of community is important for improving or maintaining health and well-being. Yet the Society is not a social club or a cult. It is the context for hard work, physical effort, spiritual nurturing and mental dedication. This holistic approach to health combines the mental, physical, social and spiritual. It gives a deeply satisfying experience and provides the opportunity for lifelong learning.

Yet the aim of the book is not to paint a rosy picture and create unrealistic expectations, certainly not of miraculous cures. The Society is not utopia, and the *Taoist Tai Chi*™ internal arts of health are not a panacea, though they help to cure many of the world's, and people's, ills.

The Society is a human institution and these arts are a human activity. Both are flawed and far from perfect, like all human institutions and activities. On the whole, though, you meet a great bunch of nice people who get along well with each other, and who help and support each other. Of course, there are tensions and frictions, misunderstandings and outbursts, 'personality clashes' and the occasional unseemly argument, but not a lot of bitchiness or political infighting. Those who find all this niceness too much to handle leave.

Others leave for other reasons. Some people come expecting miracle cures and don't get them; some people leave in frustration, their expectations, for whatever reason, not met; some people come to try out *Taoist Tai Chi™ taijiquan* and find it's not for them; some people leave because they did not realize that they would have to work so hard at it; some people come as customers to sample the wares and find that there is nothing to buy; some people come to try it because they've tried yoga, and/or boot-scooting, and/or ballroom dancing and/or Chinese cooking, so *taijiquan* is next; some people leave after the novelty wears off, or it becomes too hard, or too open-ended, or whatever. Everyone is welcome to come and free to go, as signs say at some locations.

And some people come and stay, for a while at least. One person who tells their story in this book had only been practising these arts for 5 days. Others stay for a long time, sometimes for many years, even decades. Another person who tells their story has been practising them for 25 years. In between were those who have been practising them for varying lengths of time. Sometimes some of these people speculated occasionally on why people leave, but no one tracks them down to ask them why and most don't come back to say why. These are not their stories.

Outline

These are the stories of people who have learnt *Taoist Tai Chi™ taijiquan* and other internal arts of health and who tell their stories about doing so beginning with chapter 2. They talk about their experience of learning these arts and what they have gained from them. In order to learn, there has to be teaching. Stories about teaching these arts are told in chapter 3. Not only those who are officially designated as instructors, but also those who are participants in programs tell these stories. These are not stories about teaching a move or technique, but about lessons in life, in caring and compassion taught in and outside classes. In this sense, everyone is a teacher in the International Taoist Tai Chi Society. Teaching and learning take place in the setting of a class as well, and some instructors talk about their classes and teaching them, and learning from them, in chapter 4. These instructors have trained to teach during programs at the International Centre at Orangeville and they talk about these programs in chapter 5. Participants in health recovery programs also tell their stories about participating in these programs in this chapter. Some instructors, some of whom are health professionals, others of whom are interested amateurs, talk about some of the medical or health aspects of these arts in chapter 6.

Some instructors and participants have found that chanting and meditation are beneficial and that they complement *Taoist Tai Chi*™ *taijiquan* in gaining physical, mental and spiritual benefits. They talk about chanting and meditation and their benefits in chapter 7. Master Moy initially taught these arts. He figured prominently and repeatedly in people's stories, not as a distant master to revere, but as a real force for change for the better in their lives. Their accounts of him are assembled in chapter 8. He founded the International Taoist Tai Chi Society as the context and culture in which those arts are cultivated. Stories about the Society are told in chapter 9. Chapter 10 reflects on the research for this book, including in the context of previous research on *taijiquan*. It also presents some of the observations made during the health recovery programs I attended and recorded in a journal on a spasmodic basis. Finally, it outlines some possible future directions for research into the *Taoist Tai Chi*™ internal arts of health. This book has only scratched the surface of a very rich and deep vein of knowledge and experience in Taoism, these arts and the International Taoist Tai Chi Society. It is a beginning, and as the *Tao te ching* says, a journey of a thousand kilometres starts with the first step from where we are standing now. This book is one small step in a long journey.

Two

Learning

*P*EOPLE START learning the *Taoist Tai Chi*™ internal arts of health for a variety of reasons. Some talk about their reasons for doing so in this chapter. Some are seriously ill and want to get better, or at least get no worse; others are healthy and want to stay healthy, or improve their health. A large number of those who practise these arts are somewhere between these two extremes. For many, learning these arts has also had a variety of effects, including benefits. Some people get better; some get worse; some get no worse; and some stay healthy, or even become healthier. Most people, irrespective of their condition (their health or physical condition) become fitter and stronger, more flexible, and more relaxed – and so just plain better, more healthy, human beings. When a willing participant agreed to tell their story about their experience of practising *Taoist Tai Chi*™ *taijiquan*, they began by saying why they had started doing it. One of the aims of this book is to relate people's reasons and motivations for starting, and continuing to do, it. After saying why they started doing it, they often go on to talk about the effects that doing it has had on them. Usually these are beneficial effects and these were the reasons for continuing. This chapter presents some of the benefits they have gained from doing it and the reasons for continuing to do it.

There are some common features in people's experience of learning this art. One thing that comes up time and again is the need to take responsibility for one's own health (which is why some people come to it in the first place). Another is the need to take responsibility for one's practice (which is why some people stay with it for the long term). Taking such responsibility is often regarded as important in the context of the current situation in the health sector in which people are being expected to take greater responsibility for their own health. It is also important for some people in terms of an individual journey to achieve health and well-being, physically, mentally and spiritually. These all require putting in the effort and doing the work in order to gain the benefits. The second aim and objective of the Society is to promote the health-improving qualities of this art. Practised diligently, it cultivates both body and mind to restore and maintain good health. There are no easy answers in this art, and everyone who wants to experience its benefits has to work diligently and has to start as a beginner.

This art is taught as part of an oral tradition, part of traditional Chinese oral culture. Learning takes place in a class, not alone, and not from a book or video. Information about classes and locations is available on the International Taoist Tai Chi Society website www. taoist.org, where there is also information about the history of the Society and the lineage of Taoist Tai Chi.

Faith in the long-term health benefits

Karen Evans from Toronto in Canada is an interesting 'case' because she seems to have no serious health issues or problems, but chooses to practise this art to improve her balance, flexibility and coordination, and to be energized and invigorated. This is not only for work, but also for sport. She is a healthy person who practises this art to maintain, if not improve, her health. She also does it to lessen the chance of injury when she is engaging in sport and to prepare herself better for it. Her story shows that it is not just for the sick or ill. It is also beneficial for the healthy and well. People who practise this art could be plotted on a continuum from the fit and healthy to the terminally ill, from those very much alive to those who are at death's door. Karen would be down the healthy end. Most people who practise this art would be somewhere in the middle. Karen also talks about the importance of feeling a connection between her feet and her hands in cycling and ski-ing, and about how this art helped her to do that and to make her spine stronger, not just her arms or legs. The spine is often a neglected part of the body in exercise routines and often difficult to access, engage and activate. Karen says that this art does all these things. The spine is called a column for a good reason as it is the central post that supports the rest of the body and from which everything else ultimately hangs. To exercise and strengthen the spine is to exercise and strengthen everything else ultimately. She says:

I've attempted starting practising Taoist Tai Chi[1] twice before and this is the third time. I'm 42 now and when I was 20 years old I was travelling around the world. I was in Taiwan and I practised Tai Chi with people in the central square. It was interesting that I just couldn't seem to be still long enough to take it on. Then when I was in my 30s, I came back to Canada and I tried Tai Chi again. I went through the beginners' course for a couple of months and then I tried the continuing class, but again I found I just couldn't fit the courses or the classes in with my life at the time. So I walked away from it and both times I thought that it would be really good to do this when I'm older. And then when I turned 42, I said, 'Well, you know Karen, you're older now!' And so I said, 'Let's really look at it'. So then I joined the local club.

Why I am continuing to do it is because I have faith in the long-term health benefits. I know that my flexibility is better and my strength is better. It's corresponding with two other sports that I am taking on more avidly in my life. One is mountain biking and the other is ski-ing. All three are very balance-related, like completely balance-related. So I find that an interesting thing. I find that when I do Tai Chi at the beginning of the day, I don't injure myself at all, or anywhere near as much, when I'm taking on other activities.

I think I'm much more flexible and warmed up in a nicer way, so that I react faster to other sports initiatives. I high-speed ski and

---

1 'Taoist Tai Chi' used here and hereafter by the interviewees and in the testimonials refers to *Taoist Tai Chi*™ taijiquan.

I think my reaction time's better because of doing Tai Chi, even though Tai Chi is a slower motion. I think the important things in Tai Chi for me are the feeling of balance directly in my foot and bringing those senses back to my hand, responding to the stimulus in the bottom of my foot for balance and that's exactly the same thing in biking and ski-ing – they're very focussed on what's happening in the bottom of your foot. I also just see it as a long-term goal. I see people who are 70 and 80 in very good health who practise Taoist Tai Chi and that's very encouraging.

Once I realized it was going to be a longer-term thing, it was easier for me to give myself a break and take longer to learn. This week has been really good for me for that because I see so many of the other participants who have been studying for 7 or 10, or 15 or 25 years, and that I find very encouraging because I see that everybody is still learning and still moving forward in their own space. It gives me a little courage to give myself my own space, to give myself a little break with it, instead of pushing so hard.

It's the awareness that my path of progress is mine and mine alone. I can't measure it against anybody else and so I need for my own progress to find the teachers that I can relate to or that can help me most at this time. I just need to keep practising, and I think I'm really lucky because I'm from Toronto where we have lots of really good teachers, so the impetus is on me to go and find the teachers that I need, because they may not necessarily be at my branch. I also feel like my spine is a lot stronger. It was interesting with the emphasis in the practice session on moving the spine, because I noticed at the end of it, and regularly during this week, that I've had a tired spine. I haven't had tired legs. It was only today when we started talking about it that I realized what was tired in me – it was my spine that was tired. It is a very odd feeling to think that you have a tired spine. That was just not in my awareness.

Other benefits are balance and agility, speed and response, and I think just an overall peacefulness. I think that I feel more at home in my own skin when I'm doing Tai Chi, a little more self-control doing controlled motions when I get up in the morning. I know that when I was working I would often be tired in the afternoon and, when people would normally go for a cup of coffee or a chocolate bar, I would go to the conference room to do the first 17 moves of the Tai Chi set and find that my energy level was right back up again. So I found that to be a really wonderful benefit enabling me to pull my energy back up and then actually have a proper meal. That was a better choice for my body. So that's a positive. So I find it more invigorating.

Whole body alignment

Practising *Taoist Tai Chi*™ *taijiquan* to maintain health places Karen at the healthy end of the continuum between health and illness I mentioned at the beginning of the chapter. Other people are at the opposite end, but most are in the middle. Everybody, though, usually wants to improve their balance and flexibility wherever they are on the continuum. Sometimes you can't tell from appearances where people are on the continuum, and it is only when you start talking to them that you find out that they have a condition or illness that is not visible. This condition or illness may affect their ability to practise this art, but it may not necessarily be the reason they took it up in the first place. One such person is Bill Robichaud from Jackonsville in Florida who said he has been practising this art 'for about 10 years now'. Bill is a person who has had to learn to listen to his body, to do what he can do and not overdo it. If he overdoes it, he suffers. Experiencing pain can be a part of learning this art, but basically there is good pain or discomfort when tight spots in the body associated with old injuries or poor alignment are being worked out and loosened up, and bad pain when old injuries or poor alignment are being overworked and worsened. Often it takes the eye and sensitivity of an experienced instructor to know the difference. Sometimes the movements have to be modified for the mobility-impaired.

Bill says he started practising this art because:

About 15 or 20 years before I met my first instructor and got started with it, I had seen Tai Chi demonstrated on the late night show as a use in martial arts. I was very impressed with this little Chinese man who couldn't have been more than 90 pounds or so, of fairly short stature, who must have been in his middle to late 70s. He was asked to do a demonstration and he took on 2 guys who looked to be about the size of Arnold Schwarznegger – they couldn't touch him. He just kind of moved gently and slowly and these men were just flying through the air and I thought, 'this is really amazing.' I had an opportunity for a short time on a few different occasions to take some hard style martial arts. I was never interested. I tried but I just couldn't get interested in it. But I thought, 'he's not hurting them – he's just keeping himself from being hurt.' That was interesting.

I started working in a college in Jackonsville and I heard that the year before there was a professor there on an exchange program from China who was teaching Tai Chi and I thought, 'Oh, I missed it.' And it wasn't more than a few months later that I saw advertised where there was going to be Tai Chi classes offered in the evening. As it turned out, that's when an instructor from Tallahassee started coming to Jackonsville. There was a young couple who had taken a beginners' class and were being transferred to Jackonsville. They didn't know what they were going to do in terms of keeping up their Tai Chi. The instructor agreed that, if they would get something started or arrange to have some classes taught, he would come once a week to teach the class. So in my first class the instructor asked why you're there. I told him about what I had seen – I thought this was interesting and I thought well, maybe I can learn something to which he immediately told me, 'We don't do that'. He said: 'We're doing this for people's health'. I thought: 'Well, that's a good thing too, I'll stick around'. I really enjoyed the movements. The moves were difficult.

But there was something about the class, not just learning Tai Chi, something else about the whole aura of Taoism and Taoist Tai Chi that I couldn't put my finger on, but there was an attraction there. At the time I started realizing that, as impressed as I was with what I had seen on TV years before, I was becoming more impressed with what I felt was even more powerful: the use of Tai Chi for improving people's health and helping people. That was one of my biggest encouragements for staying,.

Over the few years that I've been trying to learn, it's helped my health. I have arthritis. It gets progressively worse. It's not a problem where I'm mobile, but it is where my knees and my back, elbows and shoulders are deteriorating. I've had surgery about 4 different occasions, twice on each knee, with the surgeon telling me that within a couple of years from now (this was about 5 or 6 years ago), he claimed he'd see me back again to give me some artificial knees. I just told him, 'No. I'm keeping mine'. The recovery time was difficult but, as long as I am practising Tai Chi, it's helped me to understand alignment. I can save part of my knees a lot better now. Although I don't look at them as being really able to drastically improve, or that there won't be a problem, I know that I can retard many of the problems. I also keep them better protected. How I move is also becoming more secondary. If I keep the alignment, I don't jeopardise the angles of my knees.

I had arthritis when I started Taoist Tai Chi, but that wasn't the reason for starting to do it in the first place. Actually, when I first started doing Tai Chi and not understanding the alignment, my knees hurt more and I'd have to ice them and it was just painful and my back has always been painful. But then I wasn't aligned. I didn't know what I was doing. Tor Yus were a torture. The more I started to understand and the more instruction I received, it's now that I look forward to doing them. Tor Yus are my friend. It feels comfortable, it feels nice, to have them massage my back.

Tor Yus are a turning and stretching exercise that involves moving backwards and forwards from one leg to the other. They are especially beneficial for the hip region. They are usually taught in what is called a 'continuing class.' These classes are for students who have completed the basic beginners' course of learning to follow the 108 moves of the *taijiquan* 'set.' This takes about 15 minutes to do once you know how to follow it and about 10 to 12 weeks to learn. Aligning the body is something that others besides Bill emphasised and will came up later.

He went on to say:

> When I talk about alignment, I am talking about everything, the whole body alignment. I carry myself differently; I walk differently; I'll stand differently. It makes a difference, particularly in my work where I'm standing most of the day. It puts a big stress on the knees and back, but as a result of what I've been learning with Taoist Tai Chi, sometimes my students laugh at me when I'm teaching, not in a mean way, but they smile and they sort of get tickled because I might be talking and I might be doing a small Dan Yu or a small Tor Yu at the same time. Then I'll catch myself out and realise what I'm doing. It allows me to stay on my feet.

Dan Yus are a strengthening and flexing exercise that involves going up and down evenly on both legs. It is like sitting down into, and standing up from, an imaginary chair. They are especially beneficial for the lower back. Like Tor Yus, they are usually taught in continuing classes. As they are immensely beneficial for people with a variety of health conditions, they are also often taught and practised at Health Recovery Programs, as are Tor Yus.

Other people are in a similar situation to Bill. They come with serious injuries or conditions that mean that they have to be careful with themselves, with their own bodies. Or they have to learn to do this. Usually they have to learn to listen to their own bodies, do what they can do and not overdo it. At other times they have to learn not to listen to, or not try to do, what an overenthusiastic or inexperienced instructor asks them to do. It's all part of the training as one instructor said (and as he said Mr Moy said). In fact, this is something that can be said about every aspect of the *Taoist Tai Chi*™ internal arts of health and the International Taoist Tai Society, whether it's listening to your own body, or to an instructor you can't stand, or doing a move, or mopping a floor, or designing a website, or leading a workshop.

A while to work it in

Dee Steverson from Tallahassee in Florida has received enormous benefit from practising these arts. Like Bill, she has had to learn to listen to her own body and to do what she can do or else she suffers. Like Karen, she took a long time to work these arts into her busy schedule. However long it takes to start doing it, it is never too late, though equally it is never too early as an adult or teenager either – the sooner the better, but better late than never. Like both Karen and Bill, she talked about the importance of body alignment, particularly of the spine, which is especially important for her as she has a hereditary spinal curve. She says that she started practising these arts because:

> For quite a few years I was looking for something that was gentle to my body. I had tried jogging, I had tried aerobics and they just didn't fit the bill. They were too fast and too pounding on me. When I saw Tai Chi being done, I felt that's what I want and it took six years to work it into my busy schedule. The minute I started I knew that's what I was looking for. I expected it to be just an exercise, but after the first week I realised it was more than that.
>
> I had a very, very bad back when I started. My back hurt me so bad that I did not want to go to bed at night because I knew it would keep me awake all night. So immediately, with the very first week of Tai Chi, I could feel where it was working my back in such a way that it would be very beneficial, that it was actually helping with the pain. At the time we still did the Dan Yus and the Tor Yus in the beginner class. I couldn't wait to get off work so I could go and do my Dan Yus and my Tor Yus and my warm ups, because it would help my back so much.

Bill also talked about both Tor Yus which are a turning and stretching exercise, and Dan Yus which are a sitting down and standing up exercise. The 'warm ups', or foundation exercises, are done standing still with the arms, hands and upper body principally, though they are whole body exercises. They are taught in continuing classes too and at Health Recovery Programs.

> Sometimes these movements were very painful. Other times I would make a change. I wouldn't realise it until I would be in the middle of a set and I would go to do something, like a kick, and whatever was stopping me was not there and I'd almost fall over. It felt so wonderful because whatever it was that was tight was gone.

Helping with the back pain was not the only reason I kept coming and why I continue. I found it was a very natural movement, that it was very soothing to my body. I found a lot of the spiritual aspect. When people watch me do the set, they notice that I seem to smile because I am not usually in pain like I was before. Or if I am in pain, it's because I am working towards a goal of no pain. It is not getting worse. I know I am working to get rid of the pain. So it is a very nice soothing feeling to me.

The Tai Chi has re-aligned my body and it's slowly re-aligning my spine. We have this spinal curve that runs in our family. Of course, I got it. I can remember back when I was a small child, four or five years old, my back had started hurting then. It was something I had lived with all my life. The doctors would make it worse so I quit going to them. I did go to a chiropractor and that helped a little bit, but I wanted to do something to help my back, to help me. I felt like I should be doing something to help and so Tai Chi just fits the bill. It was just a regular beginners class. We weren't doing any Health Recovery classes, or even seated classes, in Tallahassee.

Dee was not doing anything out of the ordinary as far as *Taoist Tai Chi™ taijiquan* is concerned. She was going regularly to ordinary classes and doing normal *taijiquan* with no special exercises or techniques – and receiving enormous benefit from that. Even when people go to Health Recovery classes or programs by and large they do ordinary *taijiquan*. If they do anything different (like being helped to stand up), it is because they can't do it by themselves. This point applies as well to learning this art. She went on to say:

No one can do it by themselves, not even from a book or video. A physical therapist from a university in New England ended up going up to Toronto to meet with one of the medical advisers to the International Taoist Tai Chi Society who was also a Professor of Geriatrics at McGill University in Montreal at the time. It was during a workshop and Master Moy was there. It was quite interesting talking to that physical therapist because he had never practised Taoist Tai Chi. He had done Tai Chi twenty years ago and he thought it was marvellous. He was trying to teach himself from the book and so when he saw us doing Tor Yus he was horrified at the way we did our Tor Yus because it was such a strain on our bodies and how could you keep your balance. So he didn't understand at all that you can't get it from a book. You really can't.

Everybody needs to learn it in a class. Tai Chi is very three-dimensional and a book and a tape are very two- dimensional. At one point during the six years it took for me to work Tai Chi into my schedule the video-tapes that Toronto had used when they had shown Taoist Tai Chi on their public TV station were being shown down here on our public TV station. I tried to do it from the video and it was horrible. The first couple of moves were okay but you come to brush knees and you couldn't walk around the person to see from different angles and it was very, very hard for me to figure out what they were doing. The voice of experience here. I decided to go to a class after that, but it took me a while to work it in. It took me probably another year or two.

An enormous amount of unnecessary pain

A number of other people also say that it is not advisable to try to learn from a book or video. They are useful aids to memory for postures, positions and sequences but no substitute for face-to-face oral instruction and demonstration. Peter Turner told an amusing story about himself (at his own expense) trying to learn from a book and video. He lives in Scotland and he said:

I went down to stay with my brother who is a schoolteacher in Wales, and during the two evenings he had free during that visit, I asked him to show me the Taoist Tai Chi set. I picked up the book and the video – which I do not recommend to anyone as a way of learning, but that is what I did. I came back to Scotland and I would practise for 3 or 4 hours a day on my own. I would just work it through so I put my body through an enormous amount of unnecessary pain for the first year. I had no one to correct me and the body was not very functional. I was stupid enough in the early days, in the first six to nine months, to believe that learning from a book was okay, learning from a video was okay and that if you had enough motivation you could do it.

And then I met Master Moy. I remember the first workshop that I was in. A very good and gifted person in that workshop made a comment about books and videos not having a place in the learning process. I remember being silly enough to stand up and say that I thought they did because, if I hadn't had them, I probably wouldn't be here. I thought afterwards that it was probably not a helpful thing to say, certainly not in terms of my understanding now. That is probably an indication of quite how driven I was. I thought you could take yourself a long way. One of the things that became very apparent is that the beauty in Taoist Tai Chi is that someone else has already been along the path, and can take you there and help you to go places that you did not know were possible.

Doing attitude change

Another person who has been down the path made by Mr Moy, and who has taken her to places to which only he could take people, is Kelly Ekman, the Administrator of the Health Recovery Centre. She tells an intriguing story about her learning journey as a beginner student. Like Karen, Kelly did not enjoy the beginners' course. Some people enjoy it, like Bill and Dee; some don't, like Karen and Kelly, but they do it because they know it will ultimately be good for them, and to get to the next stage they have to complete the first stage. Like all three, she emphasised the importance of re-alignment, but not so much physical re-alignment as mental and spiritual re-alignment. All three are important components of the training in the *Taoist Tai Chi*™ internal arts of health; all three go together and work together. These arts and the Society enabled Kelly to re-align her whole life, including her priorities and situation. She says:

I started practising Taoist Tai Chi at a time when I was going through a pretty big transition in my life. I was just leaving a relationship of 20 years. I decided that it was time to focus on my own health and on my own interests. Eastern traditions had been something that I had been fascinated with for many years, since as a young child actually. I had participated in other forms of martial arts in my early 20s but not Tai Chi. At this point in my life I decided to return to it. I had started another form of Tai Chi, a Yang style form of Tai Chi, in the local community where I lived in the west end of Vancouver. I very quickly realized that it wasn't what I was looking for because it was just a physical training, and at the time I was approaching this I was very much looking at the whole package: meditation, philosophy and the foundation behind the actual physical movements. I guess that it was maybe a month after I actually started this other class that I came across the Taoist Tai Chi centre. It was purely by accident that I was walking around in that part of Vancouver. I saw the place and on the spur of the moment I went upstairs and went in. The person who was there at the time was an instructor. He introduced me to what the Society had to offer, the classes and so on, and I noticed at the time that there was a small Taoist shrine in the Vancouver club, so we started to talk about that and it was quite interesting. I knew at once that it had exactly what I was looking for. I signed up right there.

It was probably '89 or '90. I signed up and, as I do when I make decisions, I not only paid for my beginner class, I paid for a year's membership on the spot knowing full well again that this was what I was looking for. I was also going through a significant number of medical problems at the time. I had had a spinal cord injury when I was nineteen and had actually recovered quite well from it, but as you age and abuse yourself, it started to rear its ugly head again. I was in the middle of a really severe chronic pain syndrome. I had gone to Western medicine with very little satisfaction. It was a combination of things. I was living a fairly high-stress life-style, running two companies, and leaving a relationship. I had a teenage son at the time. That was also expressing itself in my physiology, in addition to the injury I was coping with at that time. To help deal with those physical problems was one of the other reasons for starting Tai Chi. What had happened because of those problems was that I was having to give up more and more of the activities I really enjoyed. My range of activities was getting smaller and smaller so I realized I had to do something about it. So I joined the Society and I started to do Tai Chi. I have to say I hated beginner Tai Chi classes because I found that it was by nature very slow with all the repetition, and I was very impatient. So the whole process of doing a beginner class gave me some real insight years later as to why people drop out and don't continue because it was very hard to go back as an adult learner. It was very hard to slow down, and it was very hard to do that repetition, but essential to get in touch.

I already knew the value of it before I came in, and I also knew myself well enough that, if I stuck with it, I would benefit from it. I have low tolerance for beginner classes in anything, whether it's in education or anything. I want to get to the meat of it, the interesting part, but you have to have that foundation first before you can get to the interesting part. I was adult enough by that time to know that if I made it through that part, I would actually enjoy it, and I did. Once I got into continuing class it was completely wonderful.

I am not sure that I immediately felt any beneficial effects physiologically. I think I was in a pretty stuck and stressed-out emotional place. Of course, being a perfectionist by nature, I don't think I really enjoyed it. I was too busy trying to make it right, but I just knew deep down that this was a very old tradition. I had done some research on it. I knew of the health benefits and I knew that if I just persisted that it would help me. I also knew that I was going through a process of sort of working on doing attitude change. I had been in this really high stress industry and was moving really fast, so this was part of the process. I think in my mind I had given myself at least a year to work on it regardless of how I felt about it, and I would make that commitment. If at the end of that time it really didn't fit, then whatever came next, came next.

That was my initial start into Tai Chi. The first year was difficult because I was also going through a break up in my life-time relationship. So I was in and out, working at it and not working at it. After that, all resolved itself. I resolved a lot of things in my personal life. I closed two of the businesses that were remaining and then went into a third business, related but different, which I did part-time. I actually chose to do it part-time so that I would have time to focus on my own health needs. I think things became a lot clearer so that the process of practising Tai Chi truly kicked in. I think that was probably in the second year I was doing it. I guess it was in '92, two years later, that I started to have other health issues. Initially we thought that they were related to the back injury, to the spinal cord injury, but subsequently I was diagnosed with MS. That was another quite dramatic event that happened at the time. It affected my vision quite severely and also I was suffering tremors which weren't conducive to the new business of photo retouching I had started doing. In those days it wasn't on the computer. It was very manual, so it was another re-adjustment and re-alignment of my life.

In the same boat

Karen, Kelly, Bill and Dee have all been practising *Taoist Tai Chi™ taijiquan* for quite a while. Even though Karen has only been doing it for five months this time around, she has had a lot of exposure to it over the past twenty years of her life. Kelly, Bill and Dee have all been practising it for over ten years each. They are obviously hooked and committed, but what about someone who has been practising it for only a few days? What are the effects on them? Kelly, Bill and Dee have received great benefit from it for their health issues over a long period. What about someone who has just started and who has a serious health issue? What sort of effects can it have on them? Can they receive benefits within a short period? One woman who wishes to remain anonymous, and who I will call Annie Watson, had only been practising it for five days when she talked about her experience at the end of a Health Recovery Program held at the Orangeville Centre. Like Dee, she did not do anything fancy or esoteric. She did the basic moves in the 'set' and the routines like Dan Yus and Tor Yus. Annie has MS and related that when she came to the Centre:

> I was in a wheelchair and I was going downhill fast because it is the primary focus of MS. After three days of Taoist Tai Chi I am in a walking frame now so I really see the difference.

Annie could walk when she arrived at the Centre, but she either chose not to, or she was advised not to, or a bit of both. The point is that, not only did these arts help her to walk, but also the International Taoist Tai Chi Society was the context that enabled her to get up and walk. Both are important. Annie went on to say that:

> My balance is so much better and stretching the right hand, which has been a real problem for me, is now a lot easier. The stretching has opened so much that I am able to do a lot more now than I ever could before. I used to walk behind a wheelchair. Now I use a walking frame.

She didn't expect that she would be using a walking frame after only three days of practising these arts and being at the International Taoist Tai Chi Society Centre (both of which are important) so she didn't bring one with her. She used the walking frame at the Centre. There is quite a story behind this walking frame as we will see in the next chapter. In fact, it has an important role to play as a prop in Annie's and another participant's stories, and almost takes on a life of its own as a character in these stories.

> I have been doing a lot of the Dan Yu and the Tor Yu and the snake. With the snake I never thought I would be able to get up again but I did, no problems. After just a few days I've used muscles I've never used before, which is great.

The snake is a move in the 'set' and an exercise that can be done by itself, either free-standing or holding on to a bar for support. It is a bit like a combination of the going down and up of Dan Yus and the stretching and turning of Tor Yus. Like them, it is usually taught in continuing classes and in Health Recovery Programs as Annie found. Although these are quite strenuous exercises, she says,

I'm not really experiencing any soreness or pain. I'm tired, but it's a good tired and I'm sleeping well.

She had also been doing the four warm-up exercises that are a standard feature of continuing classes. She did these sitting down. These and other exercises are often modified for people having difficulty with their mobility. She had also been doing a move from the 'set' sitting down. This involved turning and stretching the arms and spine, what's called 'brush knees' that Dee mentioned too. Annie hadn't really been doing anything that was specially designed for her. There were no fancy exercises, or esoteric routines. She was doing what everyone else was doing, sometimes sitting and sometimes with a bit of support on a bar. Slight modifications were made for her, but even these were the same modifications that were made for other people in the mobility-impaired group, one of whom had MS like her, another with Cerebral Palsy, another who had had a stroke, another with Alzheimer's. All of them were doing *taijiquan* seated when they needed to or standing whenever they could. Annie was working in this small group in the Health Recovery room at the Orangeville Centre with bars on the wall used for support with practising exercises and with parallel bars used for walking. She says:

Everyone is pretty much in the same boat where I am. It's really nice to be in a place and exercise with people who have different problems, but who are in the same boat pretty much. The camaraderie is great here. This has helped me gain confidence in my balance and walking. I was in a comfort zone, so it's great to be pushed. One of the other participants, Andy Ferenc, has MS, but he has less mobility than I do. He pushes me because he doesn't want me to be in a wheelchair. Because he has pushed me, it has made me have a lot more confidence too with trying different things. I never thought I would get up from doing snakes, but because he encourages me and because I can see him, I thought that if he can do it, I want to try it too. I'm glad someone else tried it first. Someone is there to encourage you. A bit of peer-group pressure goes a long way.

Supportive, non-competitive peer-group pressure is a defining feature of the learning and teaching of these arts as we will see in the next chapter where Andy will talk about how he helped Annie and how Kelly helped him.

This chapter has presented just a few of the stories about people's experience of learning these arts in Canada and the US. There are many, many more stories that could be told. Hopefully the ones presented here convey something of the richness, depth and range of people's experience of learning this art of healing, some of the effects it has had on them, and some of the benefits they have gained from doing it. These few stories have only touched the surface. They are only the tip of a very big iceberg. There are only five stories here from two countries. There are many more stories that have already been told in the newsletters of the International Taoist Tai Chi Society in the 28 countries around the world where it is active and *Taoist Tai Chi*™ *taijiquan* is practised. These 'testimonials' are powerful expressions of individuals with amazing stories to tell. A few of these will be scattered throughout the book to give an idea of their power, and of the power of this art. In the next section the first of these is presented, the truly remarkable story of Ian Shaw who has attended many Health Recovery Programs at the Orangeville Centre.

TESTIMONIAL ONE

Ian Shaw

'Just come on up'

I am from Toronto, and I am 36 years old. During Christmas Eve 1997 while most of you had visions of sugarplums in your head I had a stroke in mine. I suffered an infarction in the pons section of my brain that left me a zero-by-five hemiplegiac with dysphagia and an extreme ataxic dysarthria. In English, that means I was completely paralysed on my right-hand side. I had difficulty swallowing, and was unable to speak. I was in hospital for over four months, followed by another five in outpatient therapy and two more at a special clinic in Spain. Despite the excellence of the therapy, it plateau-ed within the year and it was very difficult for me to make any progress at all. Although my speech had largely recovered, I walked with a cane and had very little use of my right arm.

That wasn't the worst part, however. I experienced bouts of brutal depression. I plumbed the depths of depression that I could not have imagined were possible five years ago. I was morose and suicidal. I would go days without bathing or changing or getting out of bed. I would leave my apartment perhaps once a week and only then to go to the corner store. The smallest task required enormous amounts of effort. It was during one of these bouts that my family intervened. They came to my home en masse one Sunday, dragged me out of bed at four in the afternoon, sat me down and said, 'This is going to stop. We're not sure how yet, but this is going to stop.'

It was decided that I needed to be sent to somewhere. We didn't know where but somewhere where I could heal. My sister thought that perhaps I could check in to a mental health hospital. My father suggested some sort of rehabilitation centre. My brother insisted that there must be some sort of special clinic for me somewhere. There were less conventional suggestions as well. My sister-in-law is Native and thought that I would benefit from a stay at a sweat-lodge retreat she knew of. My eldest sister is a Buddhist and thought a few weeks at her remote monastery would do me some good. Then someone mumbled something about some Tai Chi place somewhere. This raised my interest; I have always been an aficionado of the martial arts, both internal and external, and it sounded like one of the better ideas to me. That is not how I wound up at the Orangeville Health Recovery Centre though.

It is a shame my mother isn't here to tell the story because it is quite poignant when she does. You see, it was my mother, bless her, that called around to these various places to find out which one would be the most suitable. Everywhere she turned she was met with:'Well, we handle depression, but not stroke.' 'We handle stroke, but not depression.' 'We need a doctor's referral.' 'We need a case history.' 'He's too young.' 'He's too old.' 'We have to interview him first.' 'We need $1000 up front.' 'There's a six-month waiting list.' And so on…

Then she called the International Taoist Tai Chi Society's Health Recovery Centre near Orangeville. Guess what they said? 'Come on up.' 'Oh,' my mother said,'but he's very depressed and antisocial…' 'Don't worry, come on up.' 'He doesn't have any experience with Tai Chi…' 'Never mind, come on up.' 'Do you need a referral?' 'Nah, come on up.' 'He's not in the best of health…' 'That's okay, come on up.' 'He has green scales and a third foot growing out of his head…' 'Just come on up.'

That sentiment greatly impressed my mother and that is how I came to be at my first Health Recovery week in December 2001. I've been to nearly every one since. I've made remarkable progress. I made progress within the first few days. My cane is at home gathering dust. I'm using my arm much more. I'm in better health, and despite reports of some surliness, in much better spirits. And in my time at the Centre I've seen the progress of others as well. These are people who have reclaimed their lives from the ravages of MS and Parkinson's, car accident victims healed, people with Osteoporosis with increased bone density, people with HIV whose viral loads are down and whose weight is up. I could go on for days, but I want to talk to you about teaching Taoist Tai Chi.

Why do we become instructors? Because our own Tai Chi improves through instruction and we get satisfaction from helping others and passing on Master Moy's gift. I'm here to tell you that if you think that helping healthy people improve their form is fulfilling, wait until you try Health Recovery, wait until you help somebody walk again. During Health Recovery weeks I have seen assistant instructors have profound insights into their own Tai Chi while helping people who need it most. It is not like any other intensive, it is an emotional experience that stays with everyone who participates. And it's only 100 bucks! Is there another week long intensive that's only 100 bucks?

I know what many of you are thinking. Many of you are intimidated by Health Recovery. You think that you need some sort of health care experience. Well, I'll let you in on a little secret: Guess what we do here during Health Recovery weeks? Tai Chi. That's it. You don't need a medical degree or knowledge of neuro-muscular disease or a secret decoder ring. Just Tai Chi and an open heart, that's it. There are two Health Recovery Instructor training weeks a year up here. Guess what we teach at them? Tai Chi.

You don't have to be a doctor or a nurse or a brain surgeon to help in a Health Recovery class. And the fact is folks – we need more assistant instructors. We need to cultivate more Health Recovery instructors and more Health Recovery classes. It is an integral part of Master Moy's vision. And I know that some of you are thinking to yourselves that you'd like to be more involved with Health Recovery but you're not sure if you have the right experience. Do you know what would happen if you were to approach Bruce McFarlane or Kelly Ekman or Mary Biddulph and say, 'I'd like to help in a Health Recovery class but I'm not sure that I have the right skills.' You know what they'd say? 'Come on up.' 'But I don't know MS from CSI…' 'Come on up.' 'But I don't know anything about anatomy…' 'Come on up.' 'But I failed grade ten biology…' 'Just come on up.' So please folks, just come on up.

THREE

Teaching

$\mathcal{F}$OR ANYONE to learn *Taoist Tai Chi*™ *taijiquan* there has to be a teacher of this art; for learning to occur, there has to be teaching; for anyone to experience benefits from doing the moves of this art, they have to learn and practise them; for anyone to go on learning, they need to teach, or to help teach, or to help in any way they can. Teaching this art is an integral part of the learning experience and of gaining the health benefits from doing it. The first aim and objective of the International Taoist Tai Chi Society is to make this art available to all. For that to happen, there has to be instructors. This chapter explores instructing and the process of becoming an instructor. It gives a glimpse of how one person became an instructor of. By enabling others to recover their health they were able to pass on its health benefits. For a health recovery story to be told, there has to be a health recovery process, and for *that* to occur, there has to be a teacher who teaches health recovery and who enables the health recovery process to occur.

Opportunities to open

In the previous chapter Annie talked about her experience of learning the *Taoist Tai Chi*™ internal arts of health for the first time at a Health Recovery Program, not only in the formal setting of a teaching session but also from Andy Ferenc, another participant in the same group. Annie spoke about how he had helped her with a bit of friendly peer-group pressure. Andy tells his side of that story in this chapter. He was able to help Annie because other people, including Kelly Ekman, the Administrator of the Health Recovery Programs and of the Centre, had helped him. He talks about that experience with Kelly. This chapter focuses on teaching these arts for health recovery. This is the case whether it is in ordinary beginner or continuing classes, or in 'seated Tai Chi', or 'special needs' classes. In a sense, everyone is in health recovery. No one is in perfect health. Every class in these arts is a health recovery class; every story about these arts is a health recovery story.

Yet the teaching of these arts does not just take place in formal classes or sessions of *taijiquan*. It takes place in the context of the International Taoist Tai Chi Society where the interactions between people and the actions of people teach others. Everyone learns from everyone else. Everyone is a teacher, not just the instructors. Bill Robichaud says, 'most people, and the Society, are my teacher.' The International Taoist Tai Chi Society is the context where the health benefits of these arts are taught and learnt, nurtured and grow. And where health recovery takes places and its stories are told.

'The Society is my teacher' is a mantra in Andy's story too. He is a regular participant at the Health Recovery programs at Orangeville, a mainstay of the Centre and very much a teacher, though he is not a formally designated instructor. He plays an important role in the mobility-impaired group encouraging and supporting other people in the group because of his experience of being at previous Health Recovery weeks and being with these people in the Health Recovery Room. He has learnt more, and teaches more, than just the physical aspect. For him, the social aspect is very important too. This involves more than idle chit-chat, but becoming and being a better, more compassionate, less self-centred and materialistic person. Andy was diagnosed with MS at the age of 42. This was a life-changing event, as was coming to a Health Recovery Program, learning these arts and becoming involved in the Society. These events and activities have challenged, and changed, him physically, mentally and personally. He says:

I had kind of neglected myself because the doctors always said, 'don't worry about it. If that's all you have at that particular age, you'll never get worse.' But they were wrong. It started to progress and started to get a little bit worse. I thought I had other concerns in my life. I guess I should have taken care of my health first before I started worrying about everything else in my life. But I decided that I had other priorities and worrying about MS was at the bottom of the list.

But my brother-in-law who had studied Tai Chi back in England said, 'you've got to do something with your life because if you don't do something, then it's just going to progress and get worse and eventually you will lose all mobility.' He had picked up a pamphlet about the Taoist Tai Chi Health Centre in Orangeville and he said, 'Here, why don't you take a look through this and give the Centre a call and maybe they might give you some information.' So I did and I heard nothing but good things so I thought I'm going to check myself in, along with my brother-in-law.

We came here for a weekend. I wasn't sure what to expect. I had not a lot of information on it. I thought that it would be something that I just probably wouldn't want anyways. It was gibberish as far as I was concerned. But lo and behold it turned out to be an awakening for me and it was probably the one thing in my life so far in the past 10 years that has changed my life. With that first visit here I have grown to appreciate some of the things that have happened to me since, since participating in the art of Taoist Tai Chi.

As far as my programs are concerned, every year I've slowly, but surely, started to increase my knowledge of Taoist Tai Chi through the various instructors. I think that everybody has an opinion as to what I should be doing and how I should be doing it, the direction I should be taking as far as my Tai Chi is concerned, a lot of fine-tuning, a lot of adjustments. The benefit that I find is that it's helped me to get out of a wheelchair or out of a chair and be more mobile.

Here's what happened with my mobility scooter when I first

came here. After coming for about 6 or 7 months of visits Kelly Ekman decided to end my adventure with my scooter. She said that if I ever came here with that thing again, that it would be taken away from me. I figured in my great wisdom that here I am in my mid 40s and somebody's going to tell me that they're going to take away my toys! So I said, 'yeah, sure.' So I took her up on it and I did bring it and within 2 days it was lost, it was gone. So I spent that whole week of Tai Chi trying to find my mobility scooter, which in reality meant that I was relearning how to walk. I did eventually find the mobility scooter. It was located at the top of a set of stairs. I thought, I'm going to show her. I'm going take that mobility scooter and I'm going to bring it back down and show her that I found it. Then I thought, you know what? That would be kind of stupid, wouldn't it? So I left it there until the end of the week.

She proved her point and that's when I started to realize what I was capable of doing and how much I had neglected myself through not walking, through not participating in a normal way. My balance was gone. Everything was not in good shape at all. But still that feeling for Tai Chi wasn't there. I didn't think that it was the key that was going to open me up as a person. I kept on coming.

What happened with the mobility scooter is they did this little thing for me and I know they did it intentionally. During one of those sessions of Tai Chi (it may have been the third day) and somehow there happened to be in the middle of the large practice hall a walking frame. I kind of looked at it. There was nobody else in the room. I kind of looked at it and looked at it and thought, 'hey, there's something new. Maybe I should try that and see how well it works.' Sure enough, I got onto that walking frame and I haven't stopped using a walking frame since. I use the mobility scooter very rarely now other than to go for a long walk with my wife. That mobility scooter is kind of in the back of my mind now. I don't use it that often. As a matter of fact, I've left it here at the Centre in case somebody else wants to use it. They can take a nice drive around if they can't get around as quickly as they would normally do.

The Centre has provided me with many opportunities to open my life, not just for myself but for others as well. I feel good about what I do here and it's a part of my life now.

It's not just the physical aspect but also the social aspect of the people that is important. That's very important to me. You have to work the body, you have to work the mind, and you have to work the soul as well. I feel that all these things combining together are helping me to open myself up as well. It's not the way I used to be, it's not the way my life used to be. Taoist Tai Chi has changed my personality in a very good way. It has changed me from being a person who was always educated to be the strongest you can be, to work as hard as you can, to provide for your family, don't worry about the other guy, try to be a success in life, try to make as much money as you can, have the best of everything you can. These are things that are basically not really natural to human beings. We pay great money to others to tell us how we should treat others and treat ourselves.

I'm starting to learn that that's just not a natural way of life. For me I'm starting to realize that there are things that come from me that are a little bit more natural. I appreciate the company of others. People who are hurt or suffering or not feeling well, I tend to gravitate towards these people. I don't know what it is. They tend to gravitate to me as well. I get a sense of being a lot closer to people. I seem to open up a little bit more as well. I have a lot more tolerance than I ever thought I had. But again this has taken me more than 4 years to be able to realize that there's another person inside of me.

If it weren't for my MS I would never have been at this stage in my life. I can say I'm a pretty lucky guy in that respect. I'm not crazy about MS of course. I've heard people say it could always be worse, and it's true, cancers, leukaemia, major catastrophes and so on. I guess I could say I'm a pretty lucky guy as far as that's concerned. There are so many new people that have come into my life. I'm starting to find a direction, more of a direction, more of a sense of who I am and that I have more capabilities than I ever thought I had. I think Taoist Tai Chi has really, really helped me.

It has helped me in opening up a little more to others, rather than just worrying about myself and driving myself to no end. Where I was going to then never led to anything. You think I'm going to be happier if I can buy a bigger car. I'm going to be happier if I can get more business. I'm going to be happier if I go on that vacation. Or I'm going to be a better person because I own this or have that. But every time that you get, the happiness is just not there. There's definitely something missing. What is it that was missing? I never knew because I thought that joy and pleasure came out of possessions. I have come to realise that possession isn't the key to it at all. It's people. Tai Chi has really done it for me. Sometimes I think about it and say, 'why didn't I do this when I was younger? Why wasn't I smarter?' It took me a long time to get to this position but at least I'm here, I'm prepared, I'm ready to go to the bitter end for this. I think if I maintain my attitude and I think if I maintain my direction and just keep on coming here to the Centre, I think I'll be a lot more successful than I ever thought I was going to be, in a very natural way, and it's a very pleasant way.

Every time I come here the one thing I do is leave my baggage outside. I come through the doors and the moment I arrive I can't stop smiling and I talk more than I've ever done in my life. I just ramble on sometimes. There are things that I say that are ridiculous, but I'm getting it out and people don't seem to mind. People are enjoying the whole atmosphere and people are getting involved. I find that I'm learning. It's taken me time. I have a whole life-time of getting rid of some of that negative stuff that would hang over my head. It's opening me up a lot more. I'm feeling more sensitive as well which is very uncommon for me. I've always thought I was more of a man's man, a tough guy and loved all the things that men do. We had a great old time, but boy the pain and suffering after all of that, but now it just lasts, all that beauty just keeps on lasting, the joy of others. I'm having a good old time, I really am, every time I come here. I'm a pretty lucky guy in that sense.

I think variety is the spice of life. We tend to go through our lives in a very tunnel-vision-like direction. I'm very, very guilty of that. I never complimented people on their achievements or reaching their goals, and I never thought it was all that important. Neither did I do it to others nor did I do it to myself. I always thought it was just a natural form. You learn things. You should be out there. You should be doing your job. I always thought people were just like me: motivated, get there, do your work, you don't need people to tell you what to do, you know what has to be done.

Now I'm starting to realize that's just not the case. Sometimes for me I find more pleasure in complimenting a person now on their achievements and goals in taking that first step, like Annie and her wheelchair. She was so comfortable in that wheelchair and then I heard that she actually walks around, not a lot. I had spoken to her caregiver when she was here and the caregiver said she occasionally walks with a walking frame at her house or behind her wheelchair. I didn't get upset, but I thought I'm going to do what happened to me. I'm going to take away that wheelchair, not that I'm personally going to take it away. I'm going to allow her to put her wheelchair away.

You know what happened the very next day? Someone had left a walking frame. The same walking frame that was left for me was left for her and she decided to try it. I had said to her, 'You've got to get out of that thing while you are here. What you do at home is your own business, but you're here now. You do walk at home. You might as well take advantage of it here. You're here for five days. Get off your arse, get behind that wheelchair and start pushing yourself around, start walking.' The caregiver was doing a lot for her as well and bringing her things and so on and so forth. She did start using the walking frame, but on top of that she got a little more involved, more Dan Yus, more Tor Yus and she was the proudest thing I ever saw with that walking frame. She was just everywhere. She would talk to you on a normal basis. It was like she never came in on a wheelchair.

Then I noticed with her she was having a hard time breathing because she used to take a breath between words and I think it was because she was sitting all the time. She said that she never did a lot of talking at home because her husband kind of anticipated and she didn't ask for a lot. Then she started chanting; she started talking more. Her lungs were getting a little bit bigger and filling more and she started to talk a lot more so she became a little social butterfly. This to me became something that I thought, 'Wow, this is a huge achievement for a person who took a giant leap forward and decided she was going to come here.' I'm sure she was looking for something to happen to her. I think through what she had done for herself, she had achieved that goal. She felt just incredible. For me that's that encouragement to help somebody to get to the next stage, the next step, the next breath that they may take. Anything I can do to help encourage that or promote that, I would truly love to do that.

It's like with Harry who had a stroke, the same thing with him. I watched him and what he was doing and things he hadn't done for a while and even encouraging him that we're going to get him a job as a greeter at Wal Mart. He'd just love that. The hand would go up and I'd say, 'Hey man, you're almost there!' It was his right arm. He had a hard time picking it up. By the time he was done here he had it up to his chest. He struggled, but boy didn't he get it up there!

Again, we always like to perform in front of others. It's always that much more pleasant when you can show somebody who's put in a lot of work into me. I really like doing that as well. People put a lot of work into me, they put a lot of time into me and I like to be able to return that by showing them that I can do it. I can work hard for this. The time that you've put into me, it's not going to waste. Also I'm not wasting any time and energy you put into me because I'm putting it to good use. I'm not going to waste it. I'm going to show you that I can do it. The best way to do it is just to perform. A lot of people come here and eventually whether they think of it subconsciously or not, it just comes out, they got to show it. You've got to put it out there. It's like anything else. If you want to learn to become a musician or you learn to become an actress or an actor, what do you want to do? You want to show it. I think that's what a lot of us do. We want to give it back and the only way we can give it back is not only to thank everyone for their energy and time, but to show you that we can do it. That's really essential for me anyway.

Andy helped Harry to perform a simple, but for him difficult, action to the best of his ability, and to increase his capability. Kelly taught Andy a powerful, but simple lesson through an action. Andy passed on that teaching and lesson to Annie. These were not lessons in *taijiquan* as such – how to do a move, where to put the hands or feet, how to do an exercise – but lessons in Taoism, lessons in life, in caring and compassion, in the quality of life, in improving Andy's and Annie's walking, their balance, their independence and self-esteem, and Harry's movement and functionality.

Time-honoured tradition

Kelly talked in the previous chapter about learning Taoist Tai Chi™ *taijiquan*. In this chapter she talks about how she became an instructor and what she has learnt about teaching this art along the way, especially to people with 'special needs' who are recovering their health, or trying to recover it. Like the lesson she taught Andy, these were lessons in learning humility and compassion. They weren't lessons in how to teach moves or techniques in *taijiquan*, but lessons in Taoism. She says:

It was wonderful in the Vancouver club, as we had an incredible amount of talent as far as instructors went. And I was very fortunate to be there. All the Continuing Instructors had a tremendous, tremendous amount to offer. I used to go to every class. I went to class almost every night and got some really incredible instruction and input. I can't remember exactly when – it was probably in that second year – an instructor came to me and asked in time-honoured tradition, 'Would you like to teach a beginners class?' Right now I can't really remember why I didn't want to teach but

I was really quite adamant about it. I didn't want to teach. I don't know whether I was feeling there was so much going on in my life at the time or what it was. I think part of it was that I didn't think I really knew enough to teach. That old perfectionist thing kicked in as though 'I don't know anything. How can I possibly teach this stuff? This is ridiculous.'

It wasn't long after that another instructor came to me and started so there was this little campaign going: 'I think you should be teaching.' Once she started asking, you might as well give in because she is not going to give up until you do, so you may as well say 'yes'. Nope, that did not work. What did change my mind was the fact that both of these two instructors were doing a demonstration up at G F Strong, the big rehabilitation centre in Vancouver. They asked this night if I would go along with them — they were doing tons of demonstrations — and I said, 'sure, I'd be happy to.'

So I went down there and, oh boy, I got hooked. I really connected with the people that we were demo-ing with because it was an interactive demo. They were trying it out. Wow! It was just so amazing how people responded to it. You could actually see people reaching out and giving help even in that short, short period of time, just in an evening of demo-ing. It was quite astonishing. That was it. Then I knew where I wanted my place to be eventually in the Society. So I thought about it overnight and I phoned up one of the instructors the next day and said, 'Well, I'm interested in becoming an instructor but,' I said, 'there's a little caveat. I'm really interested ultimately (in those days Health Recovery was called 'Special Needs') I'm really interested in learning how to teach Special Needs. I understand, of course, that I have to go through this process. I have to become a beginner instructor and learn how to teach, of course, but if there is ever an opportunity to come and assist at one of these classes or to come and do demonstrations, I would like to have as much exposure to it as possible.' This particular instructor was as non-committal as he could be. He just sort of said, 'Mm, okay', and then

I thought, 'okay, that's cool.'

In those days, even back then, we had a fairly good system of apprenticing where you would be an assistant in a class with an experienced instructor and do that for a few times until you were ready to go off and possibly teach an 'outside class' and start learning how to teach it. It couldn't have been more than a week or two later I think that he called me up and said, 'There's a class over in the north shore that's a daytime class that needs an instructor. It's a fairly good size class. Would you be willing to do that?' It's often hard to find people to teach in the day as people will be working. I was working uptown and north Van wasn't too far so I said, 'Yeah, I guess, but I really haven't done the apprenticeship. I have never taught Tai Chi. I have no idea what I'm doing.' He said, 'It's actually a good size class.' I said, 'How come so many people are coming to a beginner class in the day?' He said, 'It's not exactly a beginner class.' So my little ears went up, 'What is not exactly a beginner class?' What it turned out to be was actually a Parkinson's group and they had asked for an instructor.

So I went out there this first day and went into this class knowing absolutely nothing about anything. I came out of it practically in tears and completely mortified because I realized I didn't know what I was doing. Not only had I never taught Tai Chi before, but I had no knowledge of Parkinson's; I had no knowledge of these people's health issues; I just had no knowledge. My nature is that if I don't know something, to find out. I spent a fair bit of the time going down the mountain in panic mode. By the time I got across the water, I thought maybe I should go and find out about Parkinson's and see what there is to see. It just so happened that the Parkinson's Association had an office around the corner from the club. So as I soon as I got back to the club, I looked them up and found them there, 'oh, yay!' I went around the corner and went up and spent a couple of hours there getting information about Parkinson's and how it affected people. To a certain degree that did affect my approach to Health Recovery because I have always been intrigued with things medical, and so I really put together a lot of information about different health issues and started to study it quite intensively.

I realized that this was an area of interest. Anyone that walked in with a health problem, I would immediately start to study it. I started to look at Tai Chi from a medical perspective back then. I think my thinking has changed over the years and that will become apparent as I tell my story. I'm still intrigued with health and issues and how they affect people, but I probably approached teaching Tai Chi a lot differently then. I was thinking then that I had to understand the details of this, but I realize now, of course, that what I have to understand is Tai Chi. Understanding the details of an illness helps your relationship with the person and gives you confidence with the person, but you are not really treating that person. That's not part of it. Where I started from and where I am now is quite different. Where I will be in 10 years will probably be completely different yet again. That was when I started to become involved in Health Recovery; that was the beginning of it.

For some bizarre reason, I still have quite a resistance to teaching regular beginner classes. I think part of it was that I thought people didn't take it seriously. A lot of people were out for the flavour of the day. They'd come in and they'd be doing yoga and they'd be doing this and they'd be doing that. I think I was just overly serious about it. At the time I was thinking, 'You're not taking it seriously. Look at the health benefits. Why should I waste my time?' It was sort of silly. Over a period of time, that totally changed. I think back over those days and I was a little confused and in a different head space altogether. That was the beginning of my instruction career. At the same time of course, I was always working on my own issues and health issues.

The teacher is always learning – that is an important part of being an instructor with the International Taoist Tai Chi Society. In a way, the teacher learns just as much, if not more, than his or her students. Instructors of *Taoist Tai Chi*™ *taijiquan*, who are also instructors in Taoism and leaders of the Society, frequently make this comment.

Kelly has also highlighted the importance for instructors of knowing something about the condition of the people they are teaching, what sort of condition in general they are in, or if they have a health condition, something about it, so that they don't make unrealistic demands or have inappropriate expectations of their class. Being sensitive to people and where they are at and what they can do, is important for gaining the confidence of the student and for enabling them to do things they would not have thought they were capable of, and for gaining the health benefits of this art, not necessarily for restoring perfect health, but improving health. Certainly part of the training to be, and to continue to be, an instructor of this art is to be sensitive to people's capabilities and needs, and to try to get them to do what they can do, not conform to a pre-given idea of what everyone should look like or what their bodies should be like or what they should be doing.

A feeling of being helped

These aspects also came up when Karen Evans talks about the 'Summer Tai Chi Week' she attended. She made some observations along similar lines to these about the teaching of this art that went on there. She observed that the lead instructor taught by working with people as positive examples for everyone else to follow, but also to correct them and enable them to do things that they couldn't do, or didn't think they would be able to do. She also learnt something from *not* attending formal instruction sessions. Of the lead instructor she says:

> The way that he did it is that he brought people out of the class to have them demonstrate. Then he worked with them to improve their Tai Chi, but he was an active participant. He didn't externally criticize and he didn't use words often. He used his own body to move them, to give them the physical sensation that they needed to have. So there wasn't a sense of being criticized. There was more a feeling of being helped. That is a profound difference and the other thing is that then he would tell us what to look for, and, in fact, we could see it. So the person who was

participating was always part of the success. Instead of just being a negative example, they were the success story every single time and I found that to be positive.

It's a physical thing, so it makes sense to me to teach it in a physical fashion because, as a participant, if I can feel what it should be like, then I have a chance of replicating that. Beginning instruction isn't hands on, but they can allow people to learn using their eyes. Less words seems to be better, because it seems to confuse people less, and I think that's very inspiring. One of the things that I really appreciated is that I took an afternoon off because I was feeling unwell. I really felt that I was able to leave sessions when I was tired and needed to go to sleep. One of the things that I did appreciate is that it felt very okay just to follow your body and do what feels the right thing for you.

I found it interesting that in this group I had absolutely no qualms about leaving a session part way through or going and getting something to eat, or going to lie down, and that was a very freeing thing for me, because I was a little concerned about this class that goes from this time to this time and from this time to this time. I just can't keep up with everybody here. It was like I could fall asleep now and that was really pleasant to be allowed to do the things I needed to do. There seems to be an amount of trust that's very inspiring. The open doors, the way that it operates, the trust in people is a very nice thing, the open door policy, the pay-what-you-will philosophy, the gift shop where people pay and put the money in an envelope. I think that's a really nice thing.

I guess it translates to me in terms of having confidence in the people who are around and letting them do things they need to do. I think most people do better in an environment where there's a degree of trust for them to live up to. I just see lots of people contribute more than they would. Like it's not a hassle finding people to do dishes. People contribute. When we had to move the mattresses, people did stand up to go and move the mattresses. I think it's that circle of life and everybody giving back a little bit. That makes a big difference. Everyone gives as they can.

Not everyone can be an instructor.

But everyone can do a little bit to help. Simply 'to help others' is the fourth and final aim of the International Taoist Tai Chi Society. Compassion is the foundation of *Taoist Tai Chi*™ *taijiquan*, as the aims and objectives go on to say. It is also the foundation of the Society and it is a virtue to follow and practice. Both *taijiquan* and Taoism are important, and they come together and complement each other in *Taoist Tai Chi*™ *taijiquan* as the name implies and they function together in a group of people, a community, called the International Taoist Tai Chi Society. The complementarity of Taoism and this art is also evident in the Health Recovery classes conducted by the Society in many places around the world, and in the Health Recovery programs held at the Society's Orangeville centre and occasionally elsewhere. These are the topics of the next two chapters.

Four

Classes

*H*EALTH RECOVERY is an umbrella term that covers teaching *Taoist Tai Chi™ taijiquan* and other Taoist arts of health, such as chanting and meditation, to people with a range of health conditions or illnesses. These could be chronic, long-term, debilitating, life-threatening, or terminal – or not. Health Recovery is taught either in classes at local branches of the International Taoist Tai Chi Society, or in 5 day or shorter programs, at centres of the Society, such as at Orangeville. As the name implies, the aim of Health Recovery classes and programs is for the participants to recover their health. In many cases it is not possible for people to recover 'normal' health in the sense of regaining normal functionality and/or mobility. In these cases the aim of Health Recovery is to maintain as much as possible, if not improve, their current level of functionality and mobility, and so improve their quality of life. The aim for the participants is to get better and not to get worse. 'Do no harm' is the motto for the lead instructors and their assistants.

In the case of people with a terminal illness, the aim is ultimately, in the last words of Mr Moy, to comfort people while they are dying and after death. One of the aims of the International Taoist Tai Chi Society is for everybody to improve their health so in this sense everybody who practises the *Taoist Tai Chi™* internal arts of health is in health recovery and has a story to tell. Everybody is recovering health; everybody is in the process of recovering health. In this chapter a few people talk about

Health Recovery classes in Canada, Europe and the United States.

A position of alignment

Bill Robichaud talks about teaching these arts for health recovery in Jacksonville, Florida, in a number of different classes, none of which may have been a formally designated a 'Health Recovery Class', but in all of which there are different capabilities and different teaching emphases, designed to help the participants improve their health and their functionality in everyday life, even in such basic movements as standing up, something that many of us take for granted. Just as Bill emphasised in the first chapter the importance of being aligned for his own practice of these arts and gaining their benefits, so he emphasises in this chapter the importance of alignment for teaching his students, not only for practising these arts but also for getting them just to stand up. He has seen some remarkable results. Health Recovery stories are not only the stories that practitioners tell about themselves and their journey in these arts, but also the stories that instructors and other practitioners tell about others, and the benefits they have seen others gain. Bill says:

> At the moment I have three classes that I work, including one at a Seniors' Centre. Most of the people are between – actually they let people in at 55 – say, between 55 and late 60s. I have a class in a retirement village. We have about a dozen people in the class where their ages range from early 70s to mid/late 80s. We do the whole Tai Chi set. I have another class at the same place where folks who aren't capable of much mobility, people with Parkinson's, arthritis – severe health problems – do a sitting set. Out of those three, I wouldn't say it's a Health Recovery Class.
>
> In Jacksonville I thought maybe I would start something and see how it worked, and if anyone was interested at this Retirement Village. They had given me a call and asked if I would come out and interview with them to see if there was something I would like to offer to their residents. Then they invited me to give a presentation, so I agreed to do that. As I went in, I was figuring that

maybe 15 people would be there. I walked into the auditorium and there were about 150 people there! I thought: 'What am I going to do? I can't teach 150 people.' We talked a little bit about Tai Chi and health benefits and how it applied to them and some of their specific needs. During the presentation I asked them if they would like to do a little Tai Chi. They were all eager to see what it might be like. Since they were all sitting, I had them get to the front of their chair and talked them into getting to the point where they would be aligned to stand up. You see with a lot of older folks that, as they try to get out of a chair, they rock back and forth to get enough momentum to get up, which is so dangerous. If they don't catch themselves when they come out of that chair, they are going to eat carpet. So I talked them into a position of alignment. Once I had them there and they had their feet filled with their weight, I asked them to straighten their legs. All 150 stood straight up!

As soon as that happened I heard a lady scream from the back. I thought: 'Oh, my God, someone has hurt themselves. Oh, gosh, I've hurt somebody!' What had happened was that she was there with her husband who has Parkinson's. He stood straight up and she saw that happen and she said: 'He can't do this!' She was so excited and he just looked around and looked down at his feet: 'How did I do that, how did I get up here?' I had everyone sit back down with the understanding that they had to have a soft landing, and everybody sat down. I was excited to see something like that happen. I thought: 'Boy, this is a group of people who could use something like this – they've discovered that they understand alignment, that they can have better alignment and we can effect some real improvements in their lives. I had to keep going with it.

One of the fellows is one of the biggest sparks to the group who keeps them going. As a matter of fact, he gets them organised to meet once or twice a week when I'm not there, to practise what we have been going over and do the set. And he always has questions. He wants to know how everything is done and to get it just right. A while ago, a few months ago, he said, 'I don't know about this Tai Chi stuff and how good it is. I'll think I'll keep doing it because one thing I found out is that my suits fit bitter.' He's a character! He goes all over this place promoting Tai Chi and he's adamant to the point that he now says: 'Since we've been doing this (it's been about 2 1/2 years or so), other people have come into the village and we need to start another class.' So he was out there spearheading this whole thing. There was going to be a publicity campaign and the village was going to advertise it. It would be on their closed-circuit TV and we ended up with another class!

Build a good, strong structure

Other instructors have similar experiences of the enthusiasm of their students as they participate in the process of learning and of the joy of teaching they gain from them. Like Bill, Dee Steverson has not only received great benefit from practising the *Taoist Tai Chi*™ internal arts of health herself, but also passes on the gift to others by teaching classes, including a Health Recovery class, in Tallahassee, Florida. However, as she has received a lot of benefit herself from going to an ordinary beginners' class and not a special 'Health Recovery' class, she emphasises that 'every Taoist Tai Chi class is a Health Recovery class.' Like Bill, she also emphasises the importance of being aligned in her own practice of these arts and in teaching her Health Recovery Class. This often means getting someone simply sitting up straighter or standing up straighter. She also allows her students in this class to share their own experience, to tell their own health recovery story. She says:

I had started working with seniors in 1995 and it seemed to be a natural progression to become a Health Recovery Instructor and to go to Instructor's training programs because you get all different kinds of abilities when you deal with seniors as you do with anybody, and I could see how the Tai Chi would help them. I just wanted to learn more about how to help individuals the way I had been.

I try and build a good, strong structure and get the participants to put the weight in their bones so that they are able to either sit up straight or stand up straight so they would be able to move better. I have had a wide range of people with very minor problems and some very major problems. If they keep working at it, they have been helped – and that's the secret, it's not me doing it. They have to do it. I find pleasure in that, that it's not me that's the magician – it's the Tai Chi and the individual doing it.

I teach the exercises that are in the 'Special Needs' book published by the Society. We do warm-up exercises, we do Dan Yus and Tor Yus and then we do some exercises with the legs and the ankles just to get them stronger and more flexible. But to me the real influence, or the really important thing, is to teach the set, whether it's sitting or standing because you have all these elements, because you have all these aspects of strength and flexibility in the set. All the other stuff just builds the foundation to give the body the alignment it needs. I used just to do the set. I was talking last year to an Instructor who was saying that she found that the spiral turning of the spine was so important for her disabilities and so she kept trying to think of exercises to do with her class to turn the spine. It's just the set. It's all right there. I don't have to make anything up. I just have to teach them Tai Chi.

The benefits people gain from practising Taoist Tai Chi depends on where they come in. I think the most remarkable one I had was a lady with MS. She came in on a walker and she was very hunched up. She was a younger woman in her late 30s and within a month she had got rid of the walker and was on a cane. I couldn't believe it. It was really miraculous! Before the year was out, she had graduated and she would carry the cane with her just in case she needed it, but she was walking unaided across the floor. It was just wonderful to see that!

I worked with one lady about 30 years old who had a brain injury from a car accident and she was in a bad condition. Her short-term memory was so bad when she first started that every time she walked into the classroom she would introduce herself to me. She wouldn't know where she was and she wouldn't know what Tai Chi was. It took a year of doing Tai Chi classes several times a week before she realised and had built up a memory or made the connections back in her brain. That was about 2 or 3 years ago. She has made a remarkable recovery. She is in a regular beginning class now. She keeps taking the beginning class over and over again. She's slowly learning the moves. She smiles this wonderful smile all the time. So it's great to see that!

Some people don't really do the work. Sometimes they find it painful and they don't want to work through the pain. Some of them, I think, also are embarrassed with their going downhill, instead of getting better. So there are a lot of different combinations. I had one lady who couldn't just believe that her first class was helping her so much and she never came back again. I have the feeling that she really doesn't want to know. It's your responsibility, it's not mine. I think that's the key. I really think this is an important part of the philosophy of Taoist Tai Chi. It has given me this wonderful gift and it is up to each one of us how to handle the gift – if you can't handle it, then you do have to walk away.

What I have found is that every Taoist Tai Chi class is a Health Recovery class. I don't think we need to have this label because I have seen instructors say, 'you've got a problem, you need to go to Health Recovery' but then you have the other type of person who's on the other end and they don't want to be popped into a Health Recovery class. 'I want to be in a regular class.' You have to learn to balance it, you have to be open and that is what Tai Chi teaches us.

I would like to see the Health Recovery class expand. The potential is so great but we are lacking instructors. In my class I could have done different things if I had someone helping me. We have people who need one-on-one or two-on-one. We have to juggle people back and forth a little bit. If we could get more people involved with teaching it would be really great. We have hardly scratched the surface here. We have so many seniors in this state that we could be helping.

In my classes I'll talk about the body where some instructors won't talk about it and the lining up. Since I encourage it and talk about it, and tell them about my body and how I feel, or the experience I've had, then they'll do it too to some degree and I think that helps with part of the education.

In my classes I encourage people to open up and to share their experiences. If I initiate a conversation in the class about the effects of practising Taoist Tai Chi, they will respond and then they'll open up more doors and start talking to each other. So I encourage it. I don't tell someone else's medical history, but if they want to tell it, then it's fine. I don't encourage them to give a testimonial, but before exercising I'll say, 'My, you're sitting up straighter', and they'll respond. What I found in my classes is that people will generally talk back and forth and tell each other, not only about their aches and pains, but they'll also describe what medicines they're taking. They've become a very close-knit family. And so you don't worry about your privacy so much if you have this family feeling. If it was a very cold class and you weren't friends, then you would have more of that atmosphere of privacy.

It's also the interaction that's there that is important. What I have found is that, especially in the Health Recovery class, they look after each other. They're very loving. If somebody is missing, they'll check up on them, or if they need extra help, they'll go out of their way to help them. One of the ladies needed to go to the hospital so the other ladies were running around giving her a map so she could find her way to the hospital. They just do that. I think there is a fine line and you don't want to offend anybody. So if somebody wants to be quiet, then that's fine too.

I encourage the looking after each other and helping each other out. I see that as an important part of the philosophy of Taoist Tai Chi, not just in the Health Recovery classes, but in all classes. One thing I found, especially in the Tallahassee area – oh, I have found it in every location I've been in, unless they're having some sort of major squabble or like family conflict – that it is an extended family, it's a second family. And you know everybody's strengths and weaknesses, and we get together and we have a good time. It's home away from home, because a lot of people in this area don't have any close family. You might be from out of town, you know, moved here to Tallahassee and not have any close family, so you need somebody to be a family.

Looking for a miracle

Family is an important feature of the International Taoist Tai Chi Society that members from around the world bring up time and time again. This desire simply to help other people is evident in other Health Recovery Instructors, such as Ankie Boumans from Holland. She really likes to work closely with people and has a special gift for doing so. Like Dee, she emphasises the importance of doing, and the benefits from doing, the basic *taijiquan*. Like Bill and Dee, she retells the health recovery stories some people in her class tell about the benefits of practising this art. She says:

> I have started a Health Recovery class in Holland. I feel it's something that I can do. I've always had the ability to work with people. I was once a nurse in a psychiatric home and even then I learnt so much about dealing with people. In a Health Recovery program I found that you can be such a help for people who can't do it themselves and it's only the basic Tai Chi. They just have to work hard and do good, basic Tai Chi and that's what we learn. I've seen people who can't walk come out of their wheelchairs and walk the entire practice room. It's amazing. People who came in all bent over and at the end of the week they were standing up straight. People who were very worried and after 2 days they had a big smile and were so relaxed. It's so amazing what all this relaxation does not only for the body, but also the mind. Just 2 days!
>
> In my Health Recovery class in Holland I have, for instance, a lady, I don't know how you say it in English. We call it ME [myalgic encephalomyelitis]. It is Chronic Fatigue Syndrome. She had a severe problem. She couldn't walk further than just a few steps.

She called me and she told me that she lived half way from my home to the gym. I said, 'Okay, it's no problem. I can pick you up if you want.' Now she's doing the Tai Chi set standing up after one year. She does the entire set. The first time she could do it she almost jumped up to the ceiling! She's very happy now. She's riding a bike again. Wow, it's great! She's very happy.

I have one lady who has a severe form of diabetes. Her feet and lower legs are affected. Most of the time she walks with a stick, or for a bit longer distance, she takes a wheelchair. She hates to practice but, when she's practising, once she starts, she feels warmth in her feet and in her legs – she says, 'All right'. Also her back. She has a lot of problems, but these are a few of them.

Then I have another lady who was in a wheelchair, but now she walks with a walker. I really don't know what she has, especially not in English. I can only explain that her motor system, her muscles sometimes don't work. For instance, her legs just start twitching and she can't control that. I am working with her with some exercises and suddenly she doesn't have any control of her legs anymore and her feet start to stamp on the floor so then she has to sit down and start again after that. That's one of the symptoms, but it was that bad that she couldn't walk, couldn't dress herself. When she started her Tai Chi, she felt more relief. Now she's able to walk even without the walker. She can do Tai Chi standing now. Every week she said, 'This is so amazing because I've been in a wheelchair for almost 20 years.' It's great! It's really great. It's amazing!

Some people come with a lot of anger in their minds and, if it doesn't work immediately and they find out that they have to work really hard, they say, 'You can have that. Bye-bye'. I can't do anything about it, but explain and if they choose to leave I can't force them, and I won't. Not all the stories are whoopee, it's amazing.

I have one young girl who's in her twenties now and she has fibro-myalgia. She says, 'It keeps me on the same level so it doesn't get worse, but it doesn't get better either.' It just keeps her on the same level and she's very happy with that. So that's okay too.

I had one man, he was a very angry man, and he left because the changes weren't fast enough for him. He said he was looking for a miracle, and I said that I didn't know whether any miracles like that existed. So he left. That was almost a year ago, but a few weeks ago I heard someone say that he is coming back. So that's nice too. You can't force people, and I don't think that it's good to force people.

Trust the form

Doing basic *taijiquan* just like everybody else, or modified for people with mobility problems, is the basic aim of Health Recovery, whether it be in a Program at Orangeville or in a class in Holland or the United States or elsewhere. Helen Christian from Buffalo in New York State helps to teach a Health Recovery class in her hometown. She emphasises the importance of 'trusting the form'; from this trust the benefits will come. Like Bill and Dee, she also retells the health recovery stories of some people in the class and emphasises the power of doing the basic *taijiquan* moves in the 'set,' as well as doing warm-up exercises and Dan Yus and Tor Yus. She says:

In the Health Recovery class they have a great variety of health conditions. Some people are in a wheelchair. There's one gentleman – we don't know what's wrong with him because his mother insists there's nothing wrong with him – but he's in a wheelchair. He uses a walker and he walks very badly. We can't find out. We have people with MS. We have a woman who's grossly obese. She was one of my teachers for a while. She can't stay on her feet any longer for the set. We have people with various old age complaints and people who have broken this and broken that, replaced this and replaced that. Quite a variety.

There's one woman – she's quite elderly, about 80. She has had a variety of things wrong. I remember when she came in she was leaning on a walker. The next time she was holding on to the walker, standing up and walking. She can take a few steps by herself now. All we've done is the ordinary things, a few exercises, sitting stuff. That's all we've done. Usually the warm-up exercises rotating, turning and stretching the arms while sitting down, plus some Dan Yus holding on, Tor Yus sitting, and part of the sitting set. It works. It's very obvious when you look at her that she has positively changed. The hard part is going to be that most of the changes have taken place. They seem to have benefited. They keep coming back.

One graduated to the regular class. When he came to the Health Recovery class he told people he was 83; when he came to my beginners' class he was telling people he was 69. I heard him tell somebody the other day that he was 59.

I've learnt a lot from the Health Recovery Instructor training workshops. It's not the techniques that are important. It's the fact that you have to trust the form. I think that's really useful. It isn't any magic thing you have to know or learn to do over and above what you pick up. You trust the form. It seems to work.

People's faces light up

'Teach the form', 'do the form', and 'trust the form and the benefits will flow' is something that is emphasised by many instructors. This is the case, not just with the 'Health Recovery' classes, designated as such, but also with the ordinary beginners classes – and everything on the continuum in between. David Kroh has been teaching what he called 'a kind of Tai Chi class in a hospital.' Whether or not, like any of Bill's classes, it could be called a 'Health Recovery Class' is beside the point. It is what they do. David has been practising the *Taoist Tai Chi*™ internal arts of health for two and a half years. He is a good example of someone who has both received enormous benefit himself from practising these arts in a relatively short period and who wants to teach them and pass on the benefits in order simply to help others. He also retells the health recovery stories of some people in this class. He says:

I was helping out in the hospital in the city where I live and just to see people's faces light up when you come in and work for an hour with these people trying to do these exercises and then seeing them trying to rejuvenate and build up. It's wonderful! They just do a series of exercises. I can't do that right now because of schedule conflicts with other classes but once I get a free minute, I'll be back. I was doing it for three or four months. They were kind of long-term, health-care people. Some of them had head injuries from really bad car accidents. One lady had a problem with surgery that had gone bad and she was pretty damaged, so to speak. There was a series of people who came through the system, who were sick and were in the hospital for a few weeks, so they came to classes.

To quantify the benefits I saw Taoist Tai Chi having, would be a little bit tough. From my perspective there certainly were benefits. I remember very clearly one particular lady who had Alzheimer's. She didn't speak. She was in a wheelchair. Her healthcare worker brought her in. There was a larger group that night. She was a foreign lady. We just knew her name, but we didn't know anything else about her other than that she had Alzheimer's and she didn't speak. We were all doing exercises and there were a few people who were talking. Her worker stayed there and she was going to work the exercises with us. Out of the blue this lady started talking, mostly not very understandable. The words made sense, they were in English, but they were garbled in terms of what she was trying to say, but what really struck us was that the worker was blown away because she had never heard the lady speak, ever! Out of the blue this lady was kind of talking amongst the group and we didn't know, because it was our first experience with her, how wonderful this was. It was pretty neat.

On other levels there are people who have come to us. One particular person had a bad arm and couldn't even lift it off their lap. After working with this person for a few weeks, they were moving it quite a bit more. I don't think it was a stroke, but it was some kind of frozen shoulder. I don't know if it was a tendon or what. They really didn't have any use of it. They did everything with one arm. They were fine with one arm but they really couldn't do anything with the other one. We were stretching it out and turning it. Pretty soon they didn't have full mobility by any means or fine motor skill, but it certainly was a huge difference from what they had started with. Those are just a few examples of what I've seen.

The caring starts here at the Health Recovery Centre during the Programs. It's just mind-boggling. In one case, one of the stories I heard, I met the fellow at the end of his time here. When I heard what he went through I was in tears. It was just wonderful.

In my opinion, I don't think that there is a human being alive who couldn't benefit from it. But the reality is I look at my parents and I realize that it's not for everyone in terms of actually doing it. It seems to me that the people who are against it only realize it after they have no choice – they might get hurt or go under the knife – but if they make the decision to do this and they really work at it, they get huge benefit. They're the ones who really appreciate it. I think everyone can gain from this, and the worse the health problem, the more that it can do.

David was unable to diagnose a particular problem or condition, or to identify its cause, as these are outside his expertise, but the *Taoist Tai Chi*™ internal arts of health worked for that person because they and David trusted in the form, taught the basic *taijiquan* moves and exercises, and allowed the power of the form to produce the benefits. This is especially the case the more often these arts are practised, such as at a five day Health Recovery program at the Orangeville Centre, the topic of the next chapter.

FIVE

Programs

*H*EALTH RECOVERY Programs are the heart and soul of the *Taoist Tai Chi*™ internal arts of health and the International Taoist Tai Chi Society (and so this chapter devoted to them is the central chapter of this book). They are the place where often the most remarkable recovery of health is experienced and about which the most remarkable health recovery stories are told. These programs are made up of sustained and in-depth work on the moves of the *taijiquan* set and other movements, such as Dan Yus and Tor Yus, encountered in previous chapters. These programs are held once a month at the Orangeville Centre, though they are sometimes available elsewhere when Kelly Ekman, the Administrator of the program, and Dr Bruce McFarlane, the Medical Director, take them on the road in eastern and western Canada. They go to the core of the practise of these arts, the culture of the Society and following the Taoist virtues of exercising compassion, helping others and giving selflessly. They are also at the heart of the passing on the benefits of these arts, not only to the hale and hearty, but also to the sick and dying. The aim of the programs is not to cure illness, but to improve quality of life (especially functionality and mobility). The level of care and attention given by the assistants to participants who attend the live-in programs at Orangeville is quite astonishing. These are all core components of many health recovery stories.

Some remarkable stories emerge during these programs. One exemplary incident occurred during one program. Andreu Martinez from Spain is 27 years old and started learning these arts when he was 21. He shows that *taijiquan* is not just for old people! During the first session of a Health Recovery Program at Orangeville the whole group of participants and assistants, including Andreu, starting doing a 'set' together in the large practice hall. An elderly woman, also from Spain, sat out the *taijiquan* set after only a few moves. The lead instructor went up to Andreu and asked him to help her and take her into the Health Recovery Room with the mobility-impaired people and work with her there and do some seated *taijiquan*. She was almost 80 years old. She had had a long and tiring flight from Barcelona. The lead instructor observed that she had sat out from the set after a few moves and was attentive to her needs and situation. This level of care is one of the common features of the Health Recovery Programs at the Orangeville Centre. This is by no means an isolated incident, but a typical occurrence that shows it's a very caring kind of community. Andreu emphasised the importance of this as a part of Health Recovery Programs. Getting the right attitude so the Program is not just attending to the physical work. For him it's also the caring attitude, which is part of the spiritual side of these arts and the Society. People are caring about, and for, each other, and people are learning together and working together. Everyone does a lot of things at the Orangeville Centre together, not only the *taijiquan*, but other things as well, the chores of everyday life, such as cleaning and helping out around the place.

This representative anecdote about Andreu, the elderly Spanish woman and the lead instructor gives an idea of the atmosphere of the Health Recovery Programs and the philosophy, and virtue of caring, behind them and practised in them. Annie and Andy talked in the first two chapters about their experience of learning these arts during a Health Recovery Program. Both of them learnt these arts and had only practised them, during these programs. A lot of planning and preparation goes into these programs and the shape of them has evolved over the years. This chapter gives some background to the history and philosophy of the Health Recovery Programs by relating the stories of some key informants, and of a participant and an assistant.

These programs are the vital context for the health recovery stories of participants such as Annie and Andy.

Here's how it helps me

Judy Millen, a long time student of Mr Moy, was involved in the setting-up of the Health Recovery Program. She traces the early evolution of the Programs and retells the health recovery story of a woman she met in England that emphasises again the importance of alignment and simplicity in doing basic *taijiquan*. Judy also emphasises the importance of collegiality and collaboration in the International Taoist Tai Chi Society and the power of this and other arts, not only for regaining health for the seriously ill, but also for maintaining health for anybody who has a family history of particular maladies, or predispositions that could strike them down at any time, especially as they get older. She says:

> I was in on the development of the Health Recovery Program early on and I backed-off a bit because I felt that the planning was way too ambitious for our ability to deliver. That turned out to be the case. I wasn't the only one who felt that way by the way. The lesson we learned there was that we have to work together, that there has to be a collegial and collaborative organization for every thing, or else it falls apart. I think the way it has been happening now is kind of incremental. It's growing but there are still months that are pretty small. Then there are other times when the attendance is quite high and a lot of people are coming, well, a lot of people in terms of one's expectations. A lot of people are coming who haven't done Tai Chi. This is just astonishing. I think it fits very, very well with what might happen if we ever get involved in the Long-Term Care Facility. I was involved, but when there was a little tussle around how to get that done, I did back off a bit.

> The other piece I think that a lot of members have to come to grips with, and I finally have, is that there is only so much time in any given day. I have had to make choices about what I am going to put my energy into.

I used to come to meetings. In fact, there were some really interesting and very devoted people involved in the early start-up. A manual was written and I was asked to proofread it. There were all sorts of things that were going on that were really impressive, except that the ambition and the scope of the thing was way out of whack with the volunteers you were going to get. The other bit that was missing was knowing how volunteers actually get involved in things. Now again that blip in the Health Recovery, and it was really just a blip – it actually, in my opinion, didn't hurt us – that blip had people bringing the planning down to a realistic level. So now we have these wonderful weeks. In January-February you would find that there would be small attendances and yet people come away just lifted right up from their experience at the week. Although it's been a while since I've been, I say to people, 'Every day my script reads, 'What the hell am I doing? This is not what I wrote for my life. I've got these two jobs. One I get paid for and one I don't get paid for.' The answer here is that if you really feel you're falling off the edge, go back to Health Recovery week because that puts everything in place immediately. It just says it all in an instant.

I was in Colchester in England this summer doing a workshop. I went off to a class one morning and there was a woman called Anne in a wheelchair. She reminded me of Angelo. He has since died. His MS was spiralling down. I met a woman there whose MS I had been told was in a pretty downward spiral. I said, 'Let's get up and do some Dan Yus.' I tried to use some of the strategies that I had been taught with Angelo and they didn't work. She couldn't get up on her feet. We chatted a little bit more and then she said to Marjorie, one of the women from the club who she knew (and that was another interesting reminder – Marjorie was someone she trusted), 'Let me show you how my husband gets me up on my feet' – because Anne had told us she was doing 50 Dan Yus a day. So Marjorie comes up and puts her knees against Anne's knees and Anne grabs on – that's how she gets up. She's held back by Marjorie's knees, and so they do one of those little pully-up things. Well, I loved that, because what Anne was doing by doing her Dan Yus at home, was not demonstrating to people in her class and other Tai Chi'ers what the potential was for her, because I think you could say, 'I'm doing 50 Dan Yus at home', but people are going to look at you in your wheelchair, and know that you're having increasing physical difficulty, and think, 'No you're not'. So you need to demonstrate what you're doing. Then I said to her, she protested a little bit, and I said, 'But wait, wait! You have to teach us! We need to be taught.' She got it right away, which was very nice, because in the UK, if they're going to do Health Recovery, they have to start small with a couple of people who can say, 'Here's what I do. Here's how it helps me. Here's how I figured out how to get on my feet. Here's what you don't have to be afraid of. Here's what would be troublesome', and so forth. That again is the bottom line. This is the reason why this is so important.

The other thing I think we have to be very cognisant of at the Instructors' level, is to remind people that we can't put any science behind it, but I can be certain because I have got the gift of time here. I am absolutely the person for a stroke or a heart attack. So what we have to remember is what Tai Chi is doing for those of us who are able-bodied – the maintenance piece. Of course, again you can't get any science behind it, because you couldn't say what trajectory you'd be going in if you hadn't been doing it, but there are so many of us who know intuitively for certain that whatever the limitations – I mean, I've got a raft of stuff and none of it's really pulled me down yet, but it should have years ago. That's another thing I think somehow regular Instructor workshops should be talking about, the fact that we are maintaining stuff.

Judy provides some valuable insights into the philosophy behind, and evolution, of the Health Recovery Programs and into the way in which health recovery as a process is for everyone an integral part of the *Taoist Tai Chi*™ internal arts of health. Although Mr Moy had a vision for teaching Taoism and the Taoist arts, it was not a blueprint simply to be followed and put into practice. Things evolved, developed, grew, shrivelled, and re-grew in a different form. This was certainly the case with the Health Recovery Programs. Evolution is the keystone to the growth of the International Taoist Tai Chi Society and its activities, and not some sort of straightforward, linear development. This involves making mistakes and learning from making them. There certainly were guiding principles and an underpinning philosophy, but there was, and is, no predetermined road map. Mr Moy even said that the International Taoist Tai Chi Society would disappear if it no longer fulfilled its purpose and reason for being.

Help people to do it for themselves

Another important informant about the evolution of the Health Recovery Programs is Kelly Ekman, the Administrator of the Health Recovery Programs. She talks about the structure of the Health Recovery Program, about what you can expect if you go to one, about the processes involved in getting into one, and about what usually happens when you get there. She says:

> The program evolved. There were several attempts at developing Health Recovery Programs. There was one in the 80s that didn't quite work out. Initially when they re-opened the Health Recovery Centre it was a much more open-ended program. There was much more focus on the medical aspect. I was thinking at the time it was going to be run on a medical model and run as a medical centre. Much of the forms were designed around the concept of a hospital-intake form and out-take forms, a 17 page registration form at one point! I'm not knocking it, because the model was different, and how they'd designed it was that this Centre would be open 365 days a year and people would just come and go. There was no formal structure of a program. People would come for a week or 10 days or whatever, and whoever was there would start to work with them individually and they would be appropriate. That became very, very complex. I think after a little while they decided that that structure wasn't going to work.
>
> Then they moved onto the second part of the structure, which

was having a weekend workshop where they trained instructors, followed by an official Health Recovery week, with the thought that some of those instructors would stay on for the week and assist. At that time people started to come to the Health Recovery weeks. There were very small groups of 4 or 5 people, and that was the beginning of how this evolved. The next phase was to drop the instructor-training weekend and just incorporate the training as part of the week – just have the Health Recovery week, the participants and everybody coming together.

The structure of that has changed over the past couple of years. We're just learning, we're just learning how to manage various size groups and different groups. It's actually quite fluid now and there's a bit of continuity. Once you start to have continuity, then it evolves – if you have people changing and if you are training the people. At one point we wanted to expand it to a couple of weeks but we realized that we didn't have enough lead instructors.

The level of instruction of the lead instructor has to be quite high. They either have to have a really good knowledge of Taoist Tai Chi and quite a few years of experience at it, or they have to have Health Recovery experience, one or the other, the two go together. There were some instructors at that time who had never done Health Recovery, but who had a wonderful understanding of Taoist Tai Chi and therefore could help people with it. So the program has evolved.

First of all, the Health Recovery Program, for everyone's general information, is open to non-members as well as members. I'm the first line of contact here at the Centre. I will get calls from people who have had referrals from friends or family, and we are getting more medical referrals, actually, as well. In some cases these people may or may not have done Tai Chi. Other people call in and they're already practising Tai Chi, or they're members, or they're relatively new members. Typically what happens when someone calls in is we have a conversation and they have questions about the Centre so we talk a little bit about what the Centre does and what to reasonably expect. I get a sense of their health problems and their mobility levels and whether they need personal care, or what their needs are.

I guess one of the most important things we talk about is their goals. It's always an interesting conversation because some people are really desperate. They've run out of other medical options and they look to Tai Chi as something that can really help them. I think one of the things you have to do is to encourage people to have realistic expectations. You don't want to lead them down the garden path and say that this is a cure-all for everything. You have to have a realistic conversation based on their medical information and what they have to say.

After you're here for a period of time, you start to pick up a certain basic understanding of some of the medical conditions, and what conditions Tai Chi can help and how Tai Chi can help. In some cases, Tai Chi will help people physically and in some cases it helps heal the body. In other cases it will help slow down the disease processes, or improve the quality of life. It works on your spirit or your general feeling of well-being. It's just to try and find out a little about what the person's expectations are and what we offer. I talk to them about the week and what the structure of it is.

I just get a sense of their needs and then usually I'll send them out an information package or a registration form and when that comes back (it's not a long form anymore – it's no longer 17 pages, just two). It's designed so that the questions that are asked give us clues as to some of the things we need to ask on a second level of discussion.

One of the interesting things that does happen is that many people come here with multiple health problems. Some people will have a minor health problem that they're really working on – 'I've sprained my ankle and it's just not healing right,' or 'I've had a broken leg,' or they've had an injury or something – and they want to come back and work on it. Because that is such a huge focus, they've forgotten to mention that they've had thyroid cancer and they have heart disease – sometimes they don't even mark it down! Part of the interview process is to elicit this information as well.

Once we have that paperwork in, a copy of it will go to Ruth who is a registered nurse. I send the forms off to her. She will do a phone call and do a screening for more medical aspects. There are occasions, when I'm talking to someone or interviewing, that something will twig. I'll have a concern and I'll be able to ask Ruth, 'Perhaps you could approach this. I'm concerned about what I'm hearing here, or what I'm not hearing. Could you double-check that I'm on the right track or not?' Between the two of us we have a really good sense of where people are, whether it's emotional or medical. That's part of the process of organizing the week.

The process continues with putting together a week with whoever happens to show up and we are always pretty fortunate that the ratios seem to work out well. We've become far more adept at dealing with unequal ratios. I think the problems tend to occur when you have too many Assistants and not enough Participants. We've actually developed a program now and we can work quite well with that. Initially it was more of a stumbling block, but it's not so much of a problem now.

People who want to instruct or assist fill out a form and send it in. It's a different form. There are questions about their experience, what they've taught, where they've taught and what club they're at, which gives a sense of some of the skill levels of who's coming – over the years you get a little more familiar with the different locations and the different clubs, and who's teaching and what kind of skills they will bring. So you have that process.

Just before the week starts there's a process of sorting out the groups. Depending on the mobility levels, the groups break down. If we have one large group, we usually break down into smaller groups. There's a certain amount of mixing and matching. You sort out the groups by mobility, by energy levels and by problems of health, and then you match up Assistants who will be able to help those people. So it's a bit of a science, a bit of an art and a bit of just good luck. That's done prior to the Friday when the program starts. The final adjustments are made Saturday morning after I actually meet the people, because it is quite intriguing that, although you may have had several conversations with somebody, yet somebody will say, 'My mobility is so bad or I can't stand or I can't do this.' You take one look at the person and, of course, this person can't do that, so you may switch the group. Or you may look at somebody and say, 'Wow, that person is a little more marginal than we thought.' So you do your final adjustments that way. For the most part it works. There are occasions when you might fine-tune it during the first day or so, but generally that part of it just works. It's just practice. You get to know some of the people who come regularly; you get to know the Assistants that come regularly.

The Assistants come with a whole range of understanding and learning skills. We get people from overseas, from very young clubs; we get people from well-established clubs like Toronto, or Vancouver, or Winnipeg, or some of the larger clubs; and we get people who come from smaller locations who have very little contact with the Society as a whole. We want to bring everybody up to a certain level of understanding.

One of the most important things to remind people is that they're not here to fix other people. They can only teach what they know. That's a challenging one, because when you're in a workshop you see wonderful things happen and you see people working with people in a special way, you often assume that you have those skills yourself just by being there once, but it's not necessarily true. You remind people in Health Recovery that there are occasions when there is some touching done with people, but you have to set very strict guidelines as to how and when it is appropriate, how you interact with people and really to minimize the contact.

You're trying to teach people to help people to do it for themselves because at the end, if they can't do it themselves, they won't do it at all when they go home. It's about teaching people to be respectful; it's about giving people a sense of not being paralysed.

A really good beginner instructor can really help someone with a health problem if they teach what they understand. If they start teaching beyond their understanding, then they get into trouble and that's where most problems come. They often come when people think they know more than they do, and they don't. Part of this is just trying to educate people how to teach. A huge part of it is educating people and giving people the opportunity to look and to listen because that's the other component of Health Recovery. You can only teach what your own body understands in Tai Chi and what your own skill level is, but you also have to be able to see. We are very impatient.

You have to learn to be patient; you have to learn to watch; you have to learn that sometimes people with health problems can't do the perfect, ideal Tor Yu or Dan Yu, or anything. Their bodies can't get the perfect angles, so you have to learn what to hold onto and what to give up. A huge amount is about working together because the line between Participant and Assistant is pretty blurred. You change roles quite quickly during the week. You learn from them and they learn from you.

It's often intriguing that people who have the most astonishing changes are people who are brand new. It's just amazing how quickly they respond. I think part of it is the fact that usually an illness strikes and you have a profound episode. Then you go through a recovery period and somewhere in the health recovery period – and often with an illness you have lost some sort of capacity in your life – you realise you won't get back what you could do. You always lose a certain amount. Part of what being here at the Centre does is remind people that when they get started they really can do a whole lot more than they thought they could. Although they do have problems, although they do have restrictions, they are not as restricted in some ways as they thought. Although they are in incredible pain, the body and the mind together, when there is a will to work, is an incredible thing.

The body wants to be healthy – it wants to move. We give up movement very quickly when we have an illness or disease. Just the fact that everyone is invited to volunteer at the Centre, not just the Assistants, to do the tasks of daily living and maintaining the place. A lot of these people don't do it at home. They've stopped doing it, but they can do it. So it gives them a renewed sense of independence and well-being which also affects your health. So it's really a whole life experience. Other people come and work incredibly hard, some are marginal, so you have a whole range of people who come to Health Recovery. Some people just come for the social aspect and don't work particularly hard at Tai Chi. Just the socialising and acceptance, just the beauty and the calm of the place helps heal the spirit in a way that maybe the body will never do, but the spirit does. It crosses a lot of boundaries.

I think it is a very different thing for different individuals. It depends where you are in your life and how you approach it. It totally depends on the person's own belief system – how you approach your own life and death. For a lot of people the idea is that they are going to fight until they die. For other people it's an opportunity to come to terms and to come to peace with where they are, and to enrich whatever time they have, to have that time that is really rich, perhaps more peaceful, more quiet and more calm. I think you can only support people in a way that is appropriate. You have to respect each individual's way of dealing with their own life crisis. You can offer them a place of sanctuary, you can offer them a place of calm.

One of the things that is wonderful for people is when we have an Instructor who is qualified to lead chanting and meditation. This is very, very helpful for people who are in transition at the end of their lives. But again you have to be sensitive and respect how each person chooses to go to that place. That's very much a learning experience for everybody who is here as well.

The process for the Instructor is learning the term 'Tai Chi eyes.' I can personally remember when I started teaching and I would look at people, especially when I started teaching a continuing class. I would look at a sea of people and I wouldn't have a clue what I was looking at. It was just all these people, all this movement.

There's a skill in looking at an individual and isolating a need. There's also a skill in looking at a group and isolating a common thing that you should teach the group that would benefit everybody. There are innumerable corrections that you can give to people. The gift, and the practice of it, is to be able to find the one thing that does the most corrections with the least amount of talking. If you find one thing, it will correct half a dozen things. That's the idea. It takes a long time to do that.

It is really quite interesting when you give someone a correction. Assuming that the person is getting the correction, you should know fairly quickly if it is going to work. If the person actually does what you say and nothing happens, you have probably given the wrong correction. 'Wrong' is not the right term to use: you may have to give them three or four corrections before you get there. It takes years, it takes skill to be able to synthesise it and sort of say 'boom.'

Another big task at the Health Recovery Centre is trying to relate the East to the West, the eastern tradition to western physiology, and to understand a bit of the process both ways. That is part of the journey as well. It's quite intriguing actually.

It kind of goes back to where I started from and what I was saying when I first had my Parkinson's class. I got quite obsessed with the medical aspect of it. I think the more we understand, the more we can help, but I think we need to understand *why* we are understanding. I think it is very useful to know how people will react if their body is stressed because of the fact that they have a heart condition, or have high blood pressure, or they have cancer or are on heavy medication. These are important things to understand.

I think we want to understand them just to make sure that the person is safe, and we want to understand them so when we talk to the person we can develop a confident relationship, because, if someone comes in and says, 'I have ALS' and I say, 'Oh, what's that?' If I then tell them to stand on their head (I'm being real facetious), or go do 50 Dan Yus, this person is going to look at me and say

'Well, why do they want me to do that? This person doesn't know anything about my disease and if they don't know anything about my disease, how can I trust them and do what they are asking me to do?' It doesn't make sense.

If we are working with people with health problems it is in their interest and our interest to have some basic understanding. This information is now easily accessible. Most organizations are on the Web nowadays and most of them have incredible information that is not overly medicalized, but is in terminology that almost anybody who can read can understand. It takes a little bit of the mystery out of the disease, it takes away a little bit of the fear component, because there's a huge amount of fear working with people with health problems, if you've never been around sick people. Just having some basic understanding can relieve some of your fear.

There's nothing worse than an Instructor who's fearful trying to teach somebody, because that is immediately transmitted and translated to the person. I'm all for understanding as much as possible about a person's health issue, but by the same token you shouldn't be making any medical recommendations. What you do is understand what's happening to that person, and then you apply Taoist Tai Chi. When I look at a room full of people with health problems, I try as much as possible to understand the individual organism and the disease. When I look at a room of people doing Tai Chi, I look at the functionality of the individual person. I don't necessarily think they have cancer, they have heart failure, they have this or that. What I will look at is how's their balance, where are they tight, are they weak, are they fatigued, do they fatigue quickly.

Illness has these common qualities regardless of the health problem you have. If you went into the Health Recovery room right now you will find that half the people all share the same symptoms. The disease process and the cause are different, but they have the same problems. Why does Taoist Tai Chi work? For that simple reason. If you're tight, you need to stretch; if you have poor balance, you need to find your alignment; if you have sick internal organs, you need to get circulation; if you have poor joints, you need to get mobility.

Initially it was always a mystery. How does Taoist Tai Chi help all of this? All these people with all these different health issues, but as you start to get a little bit of a sense of physiology and understand how a body functions you realize that this sequence of movements address all of these common issues, that all of the diseases are different, but the responses, the reactions and the results are the same. That's part of how it's useful, I think.

I think the interesting thing is that we don't teach Taoist Tai Chi one-on-one. We always teach it in classes. The peer support often encourages people to do more than they think they can. If you're wise, you will put together a bunch of people who will help each other, as opposed to the Instructor always being the one who drives them. If you're confident you can set people up, and you can allay their fears. 'My knees hurt.' You can set them up in a Dan Yu that won't hurt their knees and they'll be more likely to be trusting. If you can be aware and help solve some of their small problems, they'll be more likely to trust and go forward.

Again, it's that component of the group. I try personally to avoid single disease syndrome groups because it's too closed. There's a wonderful thing that happens when you have a bunch of different people with a bunch of different illnesses getting together. They're very supportive of each other. There's a tendency that if so-and-so can do this, I can do this. It's a very positive thing. I think it's not a simple answer. You use all of these things that are at your disposal to help you. It's just a matter of experience.

When I first started I didn't know what I was doing but you try and err on the side of caution – the whole thing is you want to do no harm. Unless you're sure you do no harm, you don't do it, but as time goes on you understand what works and what doesn't work. The whole thing is experiential – it's hands on. The more you do, the more you learn, the more comfortable you become. It's just a process. When you're starting out, you teach what you understand. If you're a beginning instructor, teach the beginner Tai Chi. The form itself will help and little by little over time, if you keep at it, your knowledge and experience will increase and you'll know what to do.

The training comes by attending a Health Recovery week where you work with people who have mobility impairments and where you would go to a club and work with other experienced instructors. There is always this oral tradition, this hands-on sharing tradition. Sensitivity is something some people have, some people don't. Some people are willing to be more sensitive than others. People who are not sensitive quickly get bored with it, or it just doesn't work out. To a certain degree people are impatient to give more because they feel the need that more should be happening, I should be doing more. But very small things take a great deal of effort for people who have severe handicaps, or who are in wheelchairs, and who have real mobility restrictions. It takes a huge amount of energy to do a small movement and it is quite astonishing if someone can raise and turn their hand, which normally they can't, and then do that two or three times in a morning.

To be able to be patient and to accept that, and to encourage – that is hard actually. It is really hard to slow down and be that still inside yourself so that you can just be quiet with that person and allow them to do that. Sometimes people in what we refer to as 'the little room,' often people with the mobility problems, many of whom we see here on a regular basis, and as their health declines (which it does in time), it is a real challenge and a really interesting process as people little by little have to give up some of the things they have been doing. In some cases someone might have been doing freestanding Dan Yus, but now they have to go to the bar to do them, and then there are weeks when they cannot stand up because they are too weak. There was a time when we did a lot of physical intervention with people and we're doing less of that now because part of it is respecting where people are at and that is an important part.

Everyone supports each other

Kelly, like Judy, gives some valuable insights into the philosophy, history and workings of the Health Recovery programs. Their point of view, though, is that of an instructor and administrator, not the participant. Rachele Yerex is a participant with MS who, like Judy and Kelly, emphasises the importance of doing things together as the context in which health recovery is nurtured and health benefits are experienced. She says:

> Everything that's done is done in a group. Everyone supports each other and we just make it work. At our own club, for instance, we were celebrating our twentieth anniversary. It was a lot of work but it ended up to be really worth it just because of the cooperation. In the Health Recovery programs we do brush knees in time, do Dan Yus in time. When you're struggling with a move you can watch everybody around you, and then the Instructor stops you and you start over together. It's all very helpful for sure because there's something very helpful about doing it in a group and there are people all around you. You need each other, especially when you're learning the moves, and if you're not there and the cooperation is not there, it just doesn't happen. It helps you with your timing, and the timing's so important to get the moves so that you get the benefit from the actual move that you are trying to perform, trying to do. I am just thinking of the move that I got corrected on right now. I had no idea. I thought I had it down pat and somebody suggested I do it this way and now the move has so many benefits.

Coming back to life again

The Assistants at the Health Recovery programs tell a similar kind of story about their experience of people coming together and working together. After attending his first Health Recovery program where he was an Assistant, David Kroh noticed the way people opened up to each other and to the *Taoist Tai Chi*™ internal arts of health, both of which go together and work together. He says:

> It was pretty neat. I really had no idea what to expect. I mean, I think that's what the Society and Tai Chi are about anyway – you just kind of jump in and participate and give it your best and see what happens. Once again it was the same kind of thing. I wasn't let down by any means. I learnt a lot. It was pretty amazing to me to see that when people come in here (and they were in various states of health), they were kind of standoffish and quiet. Each and every day you can see everything building. Everybody was getting stronger and healthier, and more bubbly and laughing and just living. It was kind of like they were coming back to life again. By the end of the week everyone was in phenomenal spirits and in phenomenal shape, so to speak. Everybody made a dramatic transition in terms of their health and in terms of their mobility and so on. It was definitely eye-opening. The level of hard work that these people put in – they worked hard – but it showed in their physical development. It was definitely a very rewarding experience. I look forward to coming back.

All of these things relate to what could be called the health-recovering aspects of *Taoist Tai Chi*™ internal arts of health and the International Taoist Tai Chi Society, the topic of the next chapter. Health as a topic for discussion came up in the stories of some health professionals who practise these arts and in the stories of interested amateurs who have researched some of these aspects themselves. Before presenting these aspects, though, Peter Turner gives his testimonial to these arts.

Peter Turner

'Three strikes and you're out?

My first road traffic accident, with resulting whiplash injury, occurred in 1983 on the way to hospital. I had already had three knee operations and had been offered a synthetic patella, or just the removal of the one I had, to relieve the pain. The Kendo, Karate, mountaineering and daily road running should already have been a thing of the past. These had brought their share of injuries and contributed to the reshaping of my body. My response to this latest debilitation was the customary one of disciplining the mind to override the body's feedback, and I returned to martial training. Two further knee operations were to be required and assorted insights into the colour and taste of pain were savoured, until the mind started to make appointments the body couldn't meet.

1995

I did not start Taoist Tai Chi until late 1995, when I was already pushing 40. I felt that I had had a good run and was just beginning to think it was time to grow old gracefully.

I was fortunate to overlap in the early years with Master Moy, so he took me to some places that I may be able to find again at some stage in the future. He was able to give some really profound glimpses of what was possible for the body. So there were a number of memorable times at the International Centre and in Europe in workshops where I would describe, not in any melodramatic way, that he simply gave me experiences within my body.

Spring 1997

My knees were not working, I had 2 or 3 weeks of workshops back-to-back with Master Moy. I could hardly walk as my knee had been in excruciating pain for the first 2 years of practising Taoist Tai Chi. In the third week, we had been going for about three or four days in the workshop, it was 11 o'clock at night and the only exercise that I thought I had any sense of was the first foundation exercise. I thought I was getting some movement here (indicating rotating forearms). He came into the tearoom at Colchester and said: 'too tight – come back in the hall'. For an hour and a half he just – now I would describe it as he lent me his energy. I was just doing the Tor Yu. For an hour and a half. I could hardly walk into the room. I started doing Tor Yus on one side, didn't change, just on one side. It was some time during that experience that it felt like the spine actually dissolved. It just felt like the energy was just passing through it and I felt connected between the foot, through the spine to the head and rooted into the other foot. Now that is not the only occasion. I remember being really amazed as people came through and I wanted to just say that this is great, this is amazing. Master Moy actually had to get up off the floor and tell me to stop talking.

At the time I was always open to possibilities. I have met some really remarkable and accomplished martial arts teachers over the years, and I have seen many things that had opened up possibilities of new body and the mind experiences. But here was such a subtle, gentle thing happening. I have only experienced that sensation once since, and it was actually in a seated meditation. I happened to see, as with many other things, that it offered a glimpse of some things that might be possible. The subtlety, and creating that environment, was marvellous.

1997-98

When Master Moy came across to Europe he would often heal people in the workshop. That was always something very profound as an experience. He did different things for different people. It was very much the context for that. There always seemed to be the opportunity to establish whether someone was committed, either to working on what it was they were going to be doing, or to helping others, so I understood there was a context in which he gave. Sometimes, of course, he would give unreservedly to someone who just needed it. One of the women at the workshop was in her last days with breast cancer. He did remarkable things to her with his hands in her mouth and on her back, often what sounded like striking her really hard (he did this at other times too) and recipients of his help would say they did not feel it. There are a whole plethora of examples from different countries, of different people, but at the end, or prior to, he would always be very quiet, like the night before, gathering / purifying his energy. It was though he knew he was going to use this to heal someone. It was always something very demanding. He would always be drained afterwards. There was always something really profound.

The very first time I met Master Moy, Elliott Kravitz had already told me we had just two or three years with him, so I came quite late into this, but I still felt that it was totally amazing to me that my lifespan would overlap with somebody of this quality, and being from Western culture therefore there couldn't be any crossover at all. In my pre-university days I had always been rather attracted by the possibility of going to Tibet, or something like that, and doing disciplined study. Of course, that possibility, even if I had the language and inclination, was not real by the time I was in my 20's. It just seems to me such an amazing alignment, to have access to such a master, to overlap with his life, so there was no question but that for those years that I would spend as much time as I could around him, going several times a year to Canada or Europe. I would go to wherever he was. I began to observe that my body started to understand everything as a consequence of those early years, and I could see the transformation was going to take time and the physical work would need to be done, before I would get there.

The process of watching all that richness, the way he looked after people, including how everything was done – the caring, the serving of the meals – every aspect of the richness of the culture was just there to be observed. It was really interesting seeing it in different countries in Europe, and seeing it in Canada as well, not just to see the different techniques, but also the similarities in the approach. I really came to appreciate quite early on that it is very much more than just a physical form, and it would be two or three decades down the line before the nature of that would be accessible. It was something very different in the cultural context to experience that some profound physiological changes, witnessed in others, were starting to occur.

After two years of putting up with the pain, especially after that particular three weeks, the difference in the alignment was there, and the body opened up, and I knew right away. I was able to use the knee without popping it out at every Tai Chi class that I did. The physical benefit, which is not always manifest to everybody, was that I could walk. Originally, after the third operation, I was told by the surgeon I would either have to get around in a wheelchair, or he could replace my patella with a synthetic one, but that would be the end of my mobility. In my second workshop with Master Moy, at a monastery in Spain, I remember him just bringing a chair across in the workshop, sitting on it and asking me to do a Dan Yu and park my backside on the floor. At that stage I couldn't even sit down in a chair. He just had that way of asking me to do it. So, OK, I thought. You just let go and it happens. Some of that is physiological and trust, well it's all trust. Some things are possible and some things are a little more … I just felt the energy in the room. People seemed to be able to work in a different way when he was in a workshop.

A workshop with Master Moy was different. He just seemed to be able to balance everyone's needs. He gave instruction in all kinds of things. The classic one is balancing the food, not putting too much in, just enough, make sure that everyone had everything they needed nutritionally. It was as good to be in the kitchen as it was to be doing physical Tai Chi. So all these perceptions were there in the early part of '98, when I was here in Canada and he was deteriorating quite quickly. At this stage, with all these challenges, it was pretty clear that this was going to be something quite transformational for me. It had just enormous potential.

January 1999

The turn of year proved a significant change of fortune. I was involved in a multi-car pile-up in Kuala Lumpur in mid November. Sitting relaxed in the back seat of a taxi as I was (with a seat belt) and with a modest three years of Tai Chi I, may just have had enough health credits to make it through this one. Since my physiotherapist made me unconscious at the weekend when checking motion recovery in the neck (C6 area), I have been under the care of a neurosurgeon. The spinal cord appears undamaged and they are doing tests to eliminate problems of instability and structural damage by systematically taking X-rays of the vertebrae and using Magnetic Resonance

Imaging. The last seven weeks of headaches, nausea and dizziness have been unpleasant and, as each day has contributed to the loss of 'connection' within the organism, I have had to engage increasingly in mental games to remain in balance. I should know within the next week or two whether surgery is required – which will change my life even more materially, if not finally. Some nights the pressure in the neck is so great that I do not feel that I will endure. The upside is, I could have only a few more weeks of these severe symptoms and then a very long year immobilised in a collar.

After a new series of X rays and MRI scans last week, the consultant neurosurgeon can find no indication of bone damage and has determined that an operation will not be required – huge relief. There are a number of annular prolapses ('displaced discs') in the neck (C3/4, C5/6 and C6/7) which are causing pressure on the spinal cord. Both the consultant and physiotherapist I attend advised me yesterday to start on postural and static stability exercises, and to work through the symptoms, but refrain from Tai Chi practise. The difficulty is I need enough mobility to stimulate the circulation to clear the inflamed areas, but in the process aggravate the damaged ligaments and exacerbate the pressure and symptoms. So physiotherapy sessions always explore the limits, which are defined by nausea and pain, and subsequently reduce the quality of rest and the healing process. A good deal of my energy is focussed internally on the recovery process and I really appreciate the concern expressed by friends.

February 1999

I had my first solid sleep a couple of night's back, which is a good sign. I will be at the Colchester Centre Friday 5th to 12th. I will not be able to practise over the weekend, but hope to make myself useful and to get some advice from Dr. Elliot Kravitz during the week. I have written to Dr. Jess Goodman and intend to spend some time with him at the Health Recovery Centre. I am overwhelmed by the care and support being sent from friends in the Society as the word trickles out.

I had a wonderful experience with Elliot Kravitz at Colchester. After reviewing my assorted X-rays and MRI scans on the Friday he concluded that my neck 'was a mess' and proceeded very cautiously with sitting Tai Chi, working on the lumbar spine – with the collar as a protection. The focus was on stretching the spine, through pushing through the bubbling spring and maximising extension to open the upper thoracic area and improve the circulation to the cervical spine in particular. Over the days we progressed to increasing movement and reduced spasm. After only two painful days the lumbar area had freed up and the heat was pumping away to the middle spine. Two days later and following two modified seated sets the circulation went all the way up during a seated jong. What a joy!

I was able to appreciate the communal energy flows in the practise and learn a great deal by watching everyone practise and receive corrections. Andrew Hung and Lloyd Phillips accompanied Elliot and we had a great seven days. I shared in 10-12 hours of practice per day, working on spine alignment and observation, amongst other elements. Elliot kept a close eye on me during this time and while at rest. As I recovered I asked Elliot about timing for attempting Tor Yus and Dan Yus and which might be safer to attempt first. He replied 'The former will make you nauseous and the latter will make you blank out, so do lots of both of them.' I love his style and sense of humour!

By Thursday the collar was off. My colour had gone from white to yellow and flushed red, and Elliot shook my hand and told me that it was now up to me to 'find my own path'. Avoiding a few 'dipping the head' moves and with little stretching and sitting, I managed two standing sets without the collar and the standing jong was wonderful with the energy flowing and 'circle' complete.

It will be a long road back and Elliot emphasised that there will be some downs too, but the restoration of energy and balance, with resultant reduction in pain and tension has to be experienced to be fully appreciated. What a wondrous gift Master Moy has given us! I was so pleased for those who shared the workshop too, that they could witness the transformation. Dawn Baker provided greatly appreciated 'hands on' assistance at the start and end of programme to help relieve pain and tension. She also made the return trip to Scotland more pleasant than the trip down.

April 1999

After two weeks at Orangeville: Tai Chi week with John Huang/Chris Lewis/ Shirley Wallace, then a week as a participant at Health Recovery Centre. Help was received from Jess Goodman/Ben Chung/John Huang/Shirley Wallace/ Mary Bidulf/Peter Lambiris/Francine Laporte, together with assistants and other participants and helpers. 10 hours Tai Chi most days. Worked through several serious pain barriers to open up hips and knee, and with the chanting managed to quieten the system and relieve upper spine pain. I no longer have nausea or dizziness and pain is minimal for most activities. Left foot no longer rotates outwards. Connections are re-establishing and I am able to do more as my energy is greater and limitations are less. Circulation to cervical spine much improved with increased potential for accelerated healing.

May 1999

After a week of Lok Hup with Boon Loh in Prague – 10 hours most days. Painful neck and knee at times during practice but improved circulation, flexibility, and balance. All 'day to day' functionality seems restored and the freedom to practise.

June 1999

Fung Loy Kok week was wonderful; 'A week in the life of a monk'. We started at 8am each day with chanting and worked through Tai Chi, Sword, chanting and meditation up to 45-minute sessions until 11pm. The Ceremony for Master Moy on Saturday included 5 hours of chanting, with two short breaks, and I managed to participate in all of it. I was delighted as the nausea and pain had been rough for the two days prior – mostly due to long periods of quiet sitting and chanting with my very un-open body! Nonetheless the chest opened in a big way during the week and I am back to opening up to 180 degrees for Brush Knee etc. – which has not been possible since the accident. Karen Laughlin provided a milestone experience during seated meditation, adjusting posture with resultant sensation of 'dissolution of the spine' and the perception of using my lungs properly for the first time. The former sensation had been experienced during help with the TorYu, given to me by Master Moy in February 1997. Since the realignment I am more aware of lower abdominal compression from poor skeletal posture, so self-correction of posture has become more natural with commensurate relaxation and balance improvement.

October 1999

12 months on from the accident I have been struck down again whilst

working in the Far East, but this time by a debilitating virus, with loss of weight, blood and temperature control. I was the only one shivering in 35°C temperatures at Bangkok airport and sweating under the air conditioning unit as I endured some rough nights in Cambodia.

January 2000

After 4 months of unpleasant symptoms I made it to the Cardiff workshop. Andrew Kirby reviewed my symptoms and medication and advised me to abandon the three prescriptions that I had been taking and to concentrate on Taoist Tai Chi practice to recover my health. This has proved the start of the road back to improved health, once again.

March 2000

Philippe Gagnon has provided wonderful inspiration during his European visit in late February and early this month, in Holland, Barcelona, Colchester and Edinburgh. He pointed the way to possibilities I had lost sight of, or never glimpsed. At the end of this series of workshops my body has loosened up so much that my neck once went into spasm for a few days. This provided a timely reminder for me to work hard on recovering health, but to take the path gently and steadily.

April 2000

As this new year unfolds we have the South Wales and Edinburgh premises acquisitions and the formation of a new branch of the Society in Scotland (Aberdeen Angus), all imminent. I find myself delighted to be here to be able to be part of this exciting growth through which we can share this great gift from Master Moy.

November 2000

Warsaw (Poland) and Newport, Wales. After several days of working too hard, too intensely, my left knee has ceased to function. It had been drilled, scraped and restructured, but progress had been impressive over the first five years of Tai Chi. Tony Kwong cautioned me to walk the line [the path between the Ying and the Yang in the Tai Chi], to listen to the body and be mindful that our practice is different without Master Moy's presence.

June 2001

At a workshop in Scotland, John Huang gave me insight into alignment in the Dan Yus, helping me maintain alignment through a deep sit, with the sensation that the bottom had dropped out of the world. This was all the more remarkable as my snakes were limited to very shallow movement, due to triggering my neck into spasm or tearing adductor muscle scar tissue from an old climbing injury.

July 2001

First hands-on help from Tony with Tor Yus. I had seen him help someone in Warsaw at the International Workshop in 2000, and it looked like mechanical stretching. What I experienced was of him giving of his energy in a very precise way, to stretch tissues permanently in the body, if the instruction was maintained by diligent practice. In this particular case Tony Kwong actually physically changed the tendon length inside.

July 2002

So, over the years what I have come to appreciate is the context in which that help is given, subsequent to Master Moy's passing, over the last few years and in visits here to the International Centre: the help specifically to change my structure physically, where I had been given a correction and been working on it for a number of months and clearly not being able to do it or it was going to take a long time or if it was not going to be possible for me. More of this has come about by embracing the International Taoist Tai Chi Society which became the context for giving.

Tony offered further help to open the channels and allow alignment and stretch of the internals despite the limitations of the remaining scar tissue causing a physical misalignment. The effect was to create space inside and a sense of calmness.

As a result of this help and continued diligent practice to maintain the progress, I have been able to accept increasing responsibilities within the Society, in administration and instructional roles. These have brought a wealth of rich experiences and health improvements.

January 2004

Regular chanting, quiet sitting and a deepening trust in Society and form have been key elements in continued recovery and my ability to help others more effectively. Master Moy had said that if, in a forty-minute meditation session, you had had no thought for 5 seconds, you were making progress. So perhaps my practice is better described as quiet sitting. I certainly relate to his response to the question, 'when does the pain stop?' He replied, 'the pain goes away.' Nonetheless, the process is proving immensely useful in coping with the ever-increasing challenges to help with Society development with an ever lighter heart. This may not yet be Taoist meditation, but it provides a feeling, a sense of being 'here, now, and awake', and it's fantastic. For me the daily chanting provides a wonderful tool for pain relief and emotional re-equilibration. The path has taken me with increasing frequency into the intimacy of sharing transitioning out of the world, and these tools help me to find stillness, to centre, and manage energy depletion.

February 2004

My third road traffic accident occurred in Aberdeen just two days before travelling to Canada to lead a Health Recovery week. It has aggravated remaining damaged areas of cervical spine and pelvis, at very deep levels. Of greater concern is damage to the thoracic spine (T1-T4), triggering the cardio-pulmonary nerves in the sympathetic nervous system, with contractions around the heart especially worrying. After enduring a forty-two hour transit to Orangeville due to delayed flights, I was reminded of the exquisite nature of the pain associated with cabin pressure on the spinal cord. After three days helping with the programme at the centre and doing lots of stretching, the deep spasm was making it hard to stay centred and was providing intense pain. I tried to use the meditation but after just five minutes of quiet sitting, I endured an hour and a half of intense pain and nausea, and was once again challenged that, despite the last five years of practice and growing insight into this type of damage and using the Taoist Arts to promote healing, I was insufficiently far along the path to recover. I went into D'Arcy Street where Tony once again gave of his energy to dissipate the pain and re-align the internals. I am humbled and full of gratitude for Master Moy's gift to us, and for those who continue to cultivate this gift and use it to help others. This help enabled me to contribute more effectively to the three programmes I was involved in at the International Centre. During the week that followed, with John Huang's help, I was able to continue the focused practice required to maintain the benefits Tony had made possible. Now able to work deeper in the body I reacquainted myself with deeper scar tissue from injuries the mind had helped me forget. So John once again took me to see Tony for some further help, which he generously gave, realigning the internals and removing the pain. Tony's advice was to buy an armoured car, stay out of road traffic accidents, and smile.

In spite of the trauma, the assistants on the Health Recovery week were generous enough to observe that I still carried the peacefulness around with me and this helped others to find a quiet stillness in their practice. I find this expression of the benefits of chanting and quiet sitting a subtle but joyful gift from Master Moy, and an important aspect to cultivate to be more helpful to others.

The experience of these recent weeks has been profound and provided unexpected resonance with the help and experience Master Moy had given to me seven years before. I continue to delight in the ever-deepening understanding of Master Moy's gift to us all.

I would like to thank my friends in the Society who have helped me on this part of the path.

I offer this account as an expression of my gratitude to Master Moy for making the 'path to life' possible for me, and for giving us Taoist Tai Chi that everyone may 'add life to their years'.

SIX

Health

ONE OF the four aims of the International Taoist Tai Chi Society is 'to promote cultural exchange.' A subsidiary aim is, through *Taoist Tai Chi™ taijiquan* and other activities 'to make the richness of Chinese culture more accessible, and thereby promote greater understanding and respect among people.' This aim implies making the richness of traditional Chinese healing arts more accessible to everybody, to modern Western medicine, and to modern Western society more generally. Yet this process is a two-way street with traffic going the other way through studying and understanding the *Taoist Tai Chi™* internal arts of health in modern Western medical terms. The Society values and promotes this two-way exchange. There is a high level of interest in, and understanding of, modern Western medicine in the Society.

Mr Moy instigated the building of a bridge between the two cultures and their medical theories and practices so that there would be exchange between the two to their mutual benefit, and to people's benefit ultimately. He was personally interested in modern Western anatomy and physiology. He encouraged the understanding of *Taoist Tai Chi™ taijiquan* and other internal arts of health in Western medical terms. He appointed Western medical advisors to the Society who led workshops that focussed on these arts and on anatomy or physiology. He asked them to give lectures and write articles on these arts and on anatomy or physiology for the Society, its newsletters and its members. He was not seeking the legitimation of these arts through modern Western medicine, since it has its own legitimacy and efficacy as we have seen in all the previous chapters. Rather, he was seeking to understand, and to promote the understanding, of these arts in modern Western medical terms, and to develop the interest of Western medical and health theorists and practitioners in them. Out of this exchange a richer, broader health and medical practice has been developed, at least within the Society, for its members and for practitioners of these arts, that includes both, or the best of both cultural practices, and that prevents or lessens the incidence or severity of illness or other health conditions, and improves health. This chapter continues that legacy of his and furthers the aim of the Society to promote cultural exchange, especially in the area of health promotion and health communication.

The two previous chapters about Health Recovery classes and programs, and the two chapters before those about learning and teaching these arts, have touched on the effects of practising them, in particular on the health benefits. This chapter presents what some people, some of whom we have already heard from, had to say specifically about some of the health recovery aspects of these arts and the International Taoist Tai Chi Society. 'Health recovery aspects' refers to the health and medical aspects that were raised in some of the stories. Other aspects, such as massage therapy and brain theory, also came up and will be touched upon in this chapter.

Some of the storytellers in this book are dedicated professionals in the health and medical areas. One of them we have already heard from, and another we haven't. Bill Robichaud is a college professor of anatomy and physiology and Jacob Hunyh is a general practitioner. In their stories they discuss briefly the relationship of these arts with anatomy and physiology. They also discuss them in the context of general practice and health services. Other storytellers, such as Kelly Ekman and Dee Steverson, are interested amateurs who have read widely and thought deeply about the relationship between these arts and modern Western knowledge of the body and mind.

This chapter, however, is by no means a medical treatise and the information is not presented in Western, medical terms, nor in formal, academic prose. It gives a sense of some of the anecdotal knowledge about these arts and modern Western medicine that circulates in the International Taoist Tai Chi Society and how that informs its teaching and practice. As with many of the previous chapters, it is only the tip of the iceberg. It focuses on some aspects of the process of health recovery and understanding these arts in modern Western medical terms, in order to promote health recovery. The focus is on health, rather than medicine. The aim is to recover health, not translate these arts into modern Western medical terms (for its own sake).

This chapter also indicates the need for further medical research into these arts as is suggested more fully in the final chapter of this book. There is a large body of medical literature about research into *taijiquan* readily accessible through databases, such as Medline that lists over 300 articles in medical and health journals about *taijiquan*, addressing such aspects as balance, blood pressure, bone density and stress reduction. None of these articles address specifically the *Taoist Tai Chi*™ internal arts of health and, according to Medline, no articles about them have appeared in these journals.

Bio-mechanically correct for the human body

Bill Robichaud is a health professional who has already told his story about learning and teaching these arts. Bill is a College teacher of anatomy and physiology in Florida. During 'Summer Tai Chi Week' in August 2003 Bill gave an informal talk about these arts and anatomy and physiology, focussing on their benefits for the lymphatic system. A physiotherapist in Australia says that *taijiquan* is the lymphatic system's best friend. In his talk Bill said that lymph is a part of the immune system and that it circulates by muscle contraction. Unlike the circulatory system that has the heart to pump blood, the lymphatic system has no pump so it relies on muscle contraction alone. Yet Bill went on to demonstrate that the circulatory system relies on muscle contraction too. Bill took the lead instructor's pulse while he was doing Dan Yus and continued to do so when he stopped doing them. His heart rate increased after he stopped. For the layperson common sense would suggest that his heart rate would be higher while he was exercising, not afterwards, but Bill's demonstration showed that the circulation of blood relies on muscle contraction elsewhere in the body. The heart can't do all the work, or if it is expected to do so, high blood pressure can result. Exercising takes the stress off the heart and lowers blood pressure. The heart is not a pump like a water-pump that pumps water through the inert pipes of a reticulated system. The heart relies on other muscles to work with it.

Bill talks about the relationship between Western anatomy and physiology and Eastern *Taoist Tai Chi*™ internal arts of health in his story. In particular, and amongst other things, he says that these arts are 'bio-mechanically correct for the human body' and that it improves 'lung compliance.' He goes on to explain both of these aspects. He says:

Initially my academic background was a hindrance because I was too concerned with how does this apply. I was trying to understand it from a Western perspective and typically for someone in my field they would say, 'how does this work? Why is this working in this way?' I struggled with that for a few years and then I just let that go and figured well, it sure is doing me some good. I'm feeling better, I'm having fewer problems, so I got to the point where I wasn't as concerned with how it worked or why something worked in a particular way. I was having fun enjoying the fact that it did!

In the last few years it's been more 'it's doing good, maybe if I can get a better understanding of what's going on, then I can use this for instruction in my anatomy classes', which I've been doing. I think it is important for those folks going into the medical profession to realise that there's more to being a health provider than supplying information from a Western perspective and pushing pills. This is something that's becoming a little bit more mainstream in health providing and will become more so in the future. So maybe they'll get a little insight.

Two things did come to mind as I thought about Tai Chi and as I thought about health. One thing is that, as I make more observations, I started realizing that, as a point of view, I'm not trying to learn something new anymore. It's more I'm trying to remember. I watch my grandson. As a matter of fact I took my grandson to a retirement village where I have a class with seniors when he was just at the point where he was getting up and walking around some. I introduced him as one of my teachers, one of my Tai Chi instructors, and he nicely demonstrated a very good Dan Yu! I would watch him and I would realize that all the things we're doing in Tai Chi are things we used to do, then we forgot, and now we're going back. He was so balanced and flexible. It's nice to try and remember, and get back to that.

The other thing, reflecting on what I teach, and watching and trying to learn Taoist Tai Chi, and looking at all the moves – at least as far as I understand them – is that Taoist Tai Chi, in every way that I can find so far, appears to me to be bio-mechanically correct for the human body. I look at other types of movements, other practices, whether it's other styles of Tai Chi or yoga. Many times I would look at things about the movement or the positions, that are fine things for your health as well, but just not quite to the degree of bio-mechanical correctness that I think Taoist Tai Chi has.

As you look at the movement, at the internal structure of the movement, you can see where it comes together with all of the systems. It's not just muscle and bone. Other parts of the body come into play and are affected by the movements. Just the moving of the spine, that spiralling movement, because of the internal design of the way the organs are set up and attached inside the body, as you move the spine it will pull on the organs and cause them to massage themselves. I hadn't really thought of that for the first few years of practise, and then I started thinking, 'something's going on here', and then I realized that there was a lot more to it than strengthening muscles and improving bone density.

In my Taoist Tai Chi classes I will bring in anatomy and physiology on occasion, if it is appropriate, depending on if I'm asked specific questions and if I feel it might be useful. At other times I might gently try to move away from focussing on that and focus more on just understanding the movement and appreciating that. I do on occasion give some explanation because some of my anatomy students work within geriatric medicine. When we get to some systems, I might find certain things are appropriate to discuss with them to help them understand, for example, lung compliance. So many people breathe with just the top part of the chest. We have some very simple movements that I find to be the best thing for someone who is a little bit older and has been chest breathing all their life. They have lost a lot of lung compliance and can't really stretch to fill the lungs, so they have a difficult time even negotiating a flight of steps and breathing normally in their everyday life. There are things to give them to help stretch the lungs and give them a better quality of life.

Sometimes when they have done a movement, they may have a question because it doesn't feel like much of anything. I say, 'Don't worry about that so much. Just do the movement and think of your experience and how your body is feeling what is going on at that time'. And most people will come back and say, 'Well, gee, it seems like I'm opening up in my chest and I can breathe a little easier, but then in other parts of the movement it seems like the air is just coming out and I'm not having to do anything about it'. So instead of giving them some formal instruction, I let them think about what is happening in their own body so they can instruct themselves. You can say too much and they rely on someone else to say it. When that happens it's not theirs, it's something they've heard. It's better if they experience it themselves, they'll remember it better and they'll have a greater appreciation. That becomes more of an encouragement for them to do it on their own as opposed to saying to themselves, 'Well, gee, he told me this is good for me, so I'll have to do that'. So they're missing out on some of that.

I know that when I'd heard, 'this is good for your joints,' I was thinking of my knees in particular and all I realized at first was that my knees hurt more. But then I would get my alignment more proper, or a little bit more aligned, then I was finding it was helping me more so it wasn't so much that someone had told me. I didn't quite buy into it. It was only after I started experiencing it myself that I bought into it and I found myself doing it more – and looking forward to it as well.

Listen to the whole body

Like Bill, Dee Steverson, who has talked about learning and teaching the *Taoist Tai Chi*™ internal arts of health as well, also talks about learning more about these arts and their relationship with what she calls some of 'the medical aspects,' by which she does not necessarily mean what she also calls 'doctor medical.' She has read widely and thought deeply about this relationship in her own practice and that of her students. She mentions, like Bill, the importance of correct alignment, not only in doing *taijiquan*, but also in standing and walking. Like Karen in the first chapter, Dee talks about feeling a connection between the foot and hand in standing and moving. As Bill has just said, she also talks about learning to listen to your own body. She says:

> Slowly I am learning the names and what the different things in the body do. When I say medical, it's not necessarily doctor medical. I have been studying some things that massage therapists learn to line the body up, and learning how I can do a Tai Chi move that will help line somebody's body up, or help with whatever problem they're having. I like to take something and apply it into everyday life, combine both the medical knowledge and the Taoist Tai Chi knowledge and bring them into their lives.

> Master Moy would use the words, 'How do you feel?' I would rather use the words, 'notice what is going on in your body', because we are not trained to listen to our own bodies. One of the beautiful aspects of Taoist Tai Chi is to train you how to listen to your own body. What I've found with the Tai Chi is that usually my body will tell me what I need to do. Another reason why you have individuals doing Tai Chi a little bit differently is because they have learnt to listen to their bodies.

From some of the reading I've done on movement and how the brain affects it, I have come to realise that some people aren't aware that just a simple body movement can change the whole balance of their body. For example, if they are standing up with their feet apart and they're trying to drop their weight in the 'bubbling springs' in the front and centre of their feet, if they're aware of their body, they can feel the weight shift to the feet. Just by lifting their hand up, and dropping the hand down, the weight will shift to the toes, and just straightening the hand, it comes to the centre of the foot.

In everyday life, at least around here, you talk to people about that and you get them to do it. You really have to get them to notice what's going on. A lot of times they have trouble: 'Well, I can feel it, but I can't say it.' You say, 'Do you feel your weight shifting?' 'Yeah. That's what I feel.' So what I've found from my different research is that, with just about every aspect of the Tai Chi, you can change the weight-shift by the way you do it, even something as simple as that. And it's just the beginning.

It's a whole body experience, but you have to listen to the whole body. Sometimes my body does not want to do Tai Chi and if I stretch I'll go into muscle spasm. So I have to back off. I'll have an instructor say sometimes, 'You're not completing the move' and I know I'm not completing the move and there's a reason because if I go ahead and do it, they'll see the pain on my face. And I've done that before too. So I've had to learn to tell them, 'Not today'.

I read something just recently which was saying that, if you are noticing your movement and listening to your body, you are moving your movement from your brain stem, just the reaction part of your brain, your 'flight or fright' syndrome, and not actually moving it up to the front part of the brain, the thinking part, the awareness part. Unless you train yourself, your movements are stuck back down in your brain stem. How does that affect you? The book I was reading recently was talking about children with autism who could not speak. They found by doing simple stretching movements with these children – stretching out their calf muscles – that within two weeks they would start speaking. What they found was that the tight calf muscles on these children was affecting the angle that they were holding their spine which affected the angle that their head was sitting on their spine.

So to me something was being pinched. I found it very fascinating that it affects individuals, those particular individuals, that much – so many of your nerves come out of your spine and you might have a problem with your spine in different locations. To me, balance is very important and the spine is very important. This is what Tai Chi teaches us.

I have read *Anatomy Trains* by Tom Myers and it opens up all kinds of ideas. It talks about how you have cells in your body that add to the bones, and you have other cells that eat the bones. Depending on how your weight is in your body, if you have the weight in the bone, you add to that bone and if you don't have your weight in that bone, the other cells come and eat the bone. This was explained to me in a lecture back in the early 90s saying that if you have a heel spur, that means you're turning your foot out, all you have to do is walk with your feet straight and your heel spur will go. I didn't know why until I read this book.

There are other incidences and other things they say in that book which proves that your body was designed to heal itself. The electricity going through the bones is what makes the bones strong and yet you can move in a way so that the more weight that goes into that particular part of the bone, the more electricity the bone produces. If you don't have the weight down in the bones and you put it in the muscles and tendons, then the bones won't get it. You can really see that in the hip-bone, in the ball and socket.

One thing Taoist Tai Chi can give people who come with a terminal illness is peace of mind. I've met some people who do fit that description. They're still working and I think what it does is help them maintain what they have and give them integrity, which is fine. They don't give up completely, they have a quality of life that, if they just sat and vegetated, they wouldn't have. They're able to maintain, maybe not a complete quality of life, but a higher quality of life to the end.

I think that's important to people, otherwise some of them would be just shells and they would have to have everyone else do everything for them. I don't think we like that. But it also gives you a certain peacefulness which I can't explain. The spirit and the energy permeates and I didn't have that before. I've never heard anyone talk about it, but it has happened to me since I've been practising Taoist Tai Chi and I assume that's what's caused it.

Positive, welcoming and nurturing relationships

Giving peacefulness and creating what Jacob Huynh calls 'a nest of health' are important aspects of the health recovery process for him. Like Kelly, Jacob emphasises the importance of giving people a calm sanctuary in which to relax, and to focus and work on their own health. For both of them, the Centre at Orangeville is that place. Jacob is a General Practitioner who has been practising medicine since 2000. He takes a holistic, preventive approach to health and sees a complementary, mutually beneficial relationship between modern Western medicine and traditional Chinese healing arts, and between being a GP and a *Taoist Tai Chi™ taijiquan* instructor. He emphasises the importance of giving people a way to help themselves in order for them to take responsibility for their own health and well-being, rather than making them do it. He says:

I have a class in my practice room at the end of the day once a week. Quite a few people come to that. I also talk to my colleagues who have reservations. I recommend it for everybody, for people with lower back pain, or neck pain and then there are people with respiratory conditions such as COPD, Chronic Obstructive Pulmonary Disease – it's like emphysema or chronic bronchitis. Also for people with chronic illness like fibromyalgia, chronic pain syndrome, also for people with unstable emotional problems, depression, anxiety. I practically recommend it to everybody!

As a result they don't come to the clinic as often anymore! I have to find new clients! That's good for me. They seem to be happier and they enjoy the friends they meet in the class. I have a patient right now who has just had radiation for cancer. Normally it would be a stressful thing, but she does her exercises before she goes to the cancer surgery and she does her set. I taught her a modified Taoist Tai Chi set to do after her pelvic surgery. She did it the first day after her operation and she found that it helped her quite well. One of the things is that it keeps up her spirit because of the number of people who reach out to her in the class.

When I was young I was interested in religion and Taoism. That was one thing growing up in Vietnam we are exposed to. When I saw Taoist Tai Chi advertised in 1994 I just sat down and cried then and there. I also studied Zen Buddhism as well. That was kind of a background. Going to the Centre and seeing the people, looking at the International Taoist Tai Chi Society and the people who volunteer, and Mr Moy and so on, gives a practical way of understanding Taoism itself. It's not just in books or in discussion, but in a form where you can practically apply some of the things you read about. It's stimulating in a sense; it's not just a form of practice. It keeps making one want to learn more and look deeper.

I have been involved with meditation more than chanting, which is offered up here. Also important is the volunteer aspect, about teaching classes and drawing people together. Finding a way to help people to help themselves is very interesting to me as a health practitioner, because that's what I like to be able to share with my patients as well, not just coming to the office and treating them, but giving them a way to help themselves.

Knowledge has increased over the years and people start to get more interested in what is going on around them and how to look after themselves. You see people getting stuck into the Internet and taking a whole bunch of different herbs so there is an inherent interest in people in learning more.

On the practical level I don't know what the situation is in

Australia, but in North America, in the US and Canada, we are running very low on our resources. There always seems to be not enough doctors around to do the job. It seems to me that we can always train more doctors, but they will always be outnumbered by patients. Sometimes when people come into the office there is not enough time to spend with them as adequately as I like.

The aspect of health that is touched on is only the aspect of illness, to treat the illness rather than improve on the background of the health itself. Finding a way to improve on the characteristic of health is just as important, if not more important, than just to treat illnesses. Taoist Tai Chi gives people the chance to work on their physical health and as well as on their emotional health and their spiritual contentment. That is why I am interested in learning about it, spreading it and sharing it with other people.

We get several components of the foundations for health. We get the physical component, involving movement of the body, proper eating, proper resting, and then there's an emotional component, where you feel you are a part of the interactions in the relationships that one has that are more of a healthy nature. It could be in the family, it could be between friends. Sometimes in the office I see an emotional condition manifest as a physical condition. It could be headache, it could be migraine, it could be neck pain and back pain, but there is always an accompanying condition of things not going well in the family. It could be in their past, it could be in their present and these unhealthy things in the relationship are the things that perpetuate the illness just as much as the illness itself.

To have a place where people can form positive, welcoming and nurturing relationships, such as in a class, if we can foster that, it is as important as anything. Of course, there is the other dimension of Tai Chi in supporting health and one aspect is the intellectual part of it. The learning is there, the knowledge is there and the form and the practice are too. You can learn it your whole life and never really exhaust the knowledge, so I find that very interesting and something I like.

Then there's the spiritual aspect of things where one finds the calmness, the centring and the connection between one person and the world around. I think that is a very important aspect of health because it is the existential question that a lot of people will ask. To find a way to make a connection is of help to many people.

There are people who come and say in the class that they like themselves better. They feel like they have found inner peace in themselves. There's one 50 year-old lady who I can describe in her own words as 'like coming out of my shell.' To be able to have that kind of connectedness, you have to touch a deep core of peace inside, within oneself, and from there you can touch the world around you successfully. If we have lost the centre inside, a lot of the relationships outside may be superficial as well.

This is a long weekend and the family is around – and that is very nice – but I have had this allergy for a few days and I feel I just need a place of peace and quiet. Even though I have that place at home, it's not the same. The energy at home is different. Someone will turn on the TV and then there are demands, the phone calls – there the environment kind of reminds you of some of the things that you are yet to do. Sometimes you just have to let go of that and come to a place where you are more motivated to practice again, to practice touching that centre in yourself. Coming here to the Orangeville Centre you are able to touch that space inside again and touching that peace inside again.

In Taoist teaching there is a saying that if you treat the illness from its root, then you don't need to use a lot of force or strength or resources. If you treat the illness when it is full-grown and totally manifested, then you have to use a lot more energy and resources. A lot of the causes and roots of our diseases and illnesses are coming from misinformation, inadequate knowledge and from the structure around us, like broken families and inadequate teaching in the schools and the broken relationships we have through our lives. Things may start small, but if we continue to let them grow and build up after a while they become a problem.

For example, you can get an average student 15 or 16 years old going to high school. There may be something at home and he is not very happy. He may feel that there is no encouragement for him to go any higher with his education. Then the first opportunity comes for him after he is finished grade 11 to do physical work. Initially, and slowly, it provides him with money and means of support, and a means to prove himself and also to support the environment at home. When he goes into physical work like that he may have a body that is already physically developed. However, the knowledge of using that body is not very good, so a repetitive job and the strain that he has at work in construction or on a production line puts stress on to the back, neck and shoulders. He starts to have a problem with back pain, neck pain, tendonitis, and then we get into a problem of illness, which may become longer than expected, because with the illness he may miss work and, missing work, there is lack of income or poorer income, and then they connect maybe with disharmony in the family at home with his wife or something like that. Sometimes they want to go back to work before they are ready and relearn the skills. It sets the stage for re-injuring their back and neck. After a few times like that the person is so broken physically, and also exhausted emotionally and spiritually, because the breadwinner is not able to win anymore bread and they have to survive on unemployment benefits – in the later stages it could be welfare or a disability pension. A lot of time they don't grant disability.

I am involved in trying to find disability for a few of my patients right now. It's not easy to get and disability doesn't give you very much support. That's the story of how a person gets to 35 years old and now is labelled disabled and useless. That sets the stage for how are you going to continue to raise up children and continue to function in the family as a husband and a father. That sets the stage for, let's say, depression and for other problems that are going on. If we just have a little bit of background in the family, it might set the stage for alcoholism. The misinformation and the emotional stuff that we have in our family and in our school contributes too. A lot of the time in school children are competing with each other for knowledge and for other things like fashion. It's kind of a cycle that we set for other people and ourselves. That kind of misknowledge and misinformation, the poor support we create for ourselves, bring us to where suddenly we wake up and we are in a mess.

If that person who had left school at 15 or 16 and went to work in construction or production had started Taoist Tai Chi at that time, they would tell a different life-story. When we start in Taoist Tai Chi the body will be more flexible, more properly aligned. There is a technique that we use that is inherent in learning the set of Taoist Tai Chi where it could be structurally strong for the physical work that they do. Working in the Society or practising it the first aspect they learn about is helping themselves in the physical body. It also helps them in finding that, if you go to a class and become a teacher, then there's that emotional connection with other people around as well. A lot of the time I get a call just before I go to class, but I know if I go to class I feel better after that.

Just being surrounded by a group of people – they don't have to say anything to you – just their harmonious presence is enough to strengthen you up. If he did it alone he would have a harder time, but if he relied on the strength of the group, the strength of the class, then he would learn something that is very helpful, very valuable. It cannot be put into financial terms, but it is something that can bring him over the hump if he has problems at work – if he has an argument with a colleague, a co-worker, he doesn't feel so angry, which we know is related to tension and can predispose people to get into various problems with their spine. We can say that a lot of tension in the spine can cause more injury as well. If he successfully lasts for long he may be a teacher in the art, an instructor, and then he can feel his value as more than just a breadwinner and somehow help other people in attaining better health. Slowly by learning, by giving, it can create this nest of health that can strengthen the person.

Number one, we are talking about a group where we know for sure that, if in Taoist Tai Chi we create a welcoming environment, anybody who sticks on long with Taoist Tai Chi will benefit. It doesn't matter where they start from, who they are or what level they start at. If they stay long enough, they will get the benefit. I think the task of each class is to create a welcoming environment so that people stick and stay and learn. If we were sure to have a thing like that in the class, the person who comes with depression, the first thing I think they will find is some form of calmness in themselves because now they have something beyond their mind to focus on, something more concrete, that is their body, and how it is positioned in space, the hand, the feet, the spine. Just paying attention to that will give people a period of rest from all the wool-gathering that they have going on inside their heads.

People come to the first one or two classes and they sleep better because they don't have to think about their lack of sleep all the time anymore. I think for those people the meditative aspect of Taoist Tai Chi actually kicks-in very fast. The physical strengthening is there, the balance, the alignment. They are aware of their body more. People who are depressed get sick more often too because of some decrease with their immune system. When the body becomes stronger they start to talk about that they don't get as cold anymore, or they sleep better, or they might have a better appetite. People say they are not always hungry and don't gain weight, they don't have a good appetite but now they say that they start to have a better appetite. That's the kind of thing that they start to notice with themselves.

Some people say that they start to smile more because that is one thing we ask people to do – to smile when they come and practise – to relax their jaw. You know in our culture they talk about keeping a stiff upper lip so everybody has constant tension in their face until we tell people to drop it now and smile. They relax the jaw and muscles in the face. They start to be open more and to talk more. Give it enough time to be able to reach out to other people and to make discussion, to make a connection, to have a conversation. These times in Tai Chi are very important, to give people a chance to rest and relax and to make friends, to reach out and to come out of their shell a little. Hopefully, within the class there will be one or two people that they feel they can share things with and be connected to. These little friendships are not competitive. People start to see a different light on their situation. Perhaps their situation has not changed, but now they have the strength to carry it through. People will see that the strength they've found in the physical part will permeate into their character. They can take it more calmly.

One of the students in my class said that after he learnt it for a year the road rage just disappeared. That's a good effect, not only for him, but also for anybody who has to share the road with him!

We need a change in environment to help us reach that inner stillness more easily. Some are easier than others. One of the benefits of a Centre like this is it can be more than a regular class. You have more time to devote just to your own practice. For people who have severe illness, a short period of time is helpful, but probably not adequate. If you are very ill, you need that 100% attention to your own health and it's very hard to get that in your own house. It's very hard to give attention to improving your own health, but to come here and let go of those concerns and worries and to just spend time devoted 100% to healing I think is so important.

The aspect of seeing people who are in similar shoes, seeing what they are going through or what they have gone through before, gives you hope, gives you courage as well as nurturing some part of yourself. Touching that calmness inside yourself takes some time, some appropriate condition like an environment, like people welcoming, or meditative practice, like we do, with chanting or sitting meditation. Sometimes you have to do it seven days in a row to really touch it. If you mix dirt in a cup of water, it takes several hours or days for the dirt to settle and the water to become clear on top. Sometimes we need that extended period of time to clear ourselves so we don't have to react to things around us, stay where we can be centred and respond appropriately to whatever demands there are.

The food is good. I certainly come here for the food.

It's a practice. You have to practice it; you have to taste it. It is not anything you can see from the outside. You hear people talk about it. It's rather like looking at a menu without tasting the food. People who want to know, need to taste it for themselves. They can have a real experience when they do that. The book is like the menu.

The next item on the menu is chanting and meditation, an integral part of the health recovery process, and programs, which is important for alignment and pain relief and not some esoteric and mysterious practice. Before that, though, Helen Gaunt gives her testimonial to the *Taoist Tai Chi*™ internal arts of health. Her story is one of the major inspirations for researching and writing this book.

Helen Gaunt

A testimonial to Taoist Tai Chi

My Tai Chi life started about 10 years ago after a diagnosis of thyroid cancer. Although discovered early enough and not likely to be fatal, after undergoing treatment I set about the path of improving my lifestyle. Thanks to Sandra and Rodney Giblett being my catalyst, I was able to get going. I can honestly say I didn't enjoy it much in the early days as I had to learn to still the mind something at which I had never been very good. But with time, persistence and encouragement from Linde Millett-Beatie, my instructor, I keep going.

It was at the end of my first year in 1994 that I went to a Master Moy Workshop. I met this humble man who had given us so much and I was hooked. I hoped I could become an instructor and help others too. Over the years I have attended many workshops and met many wonderful people. At one workshop Elliot Kravitz spoke on how practising Taoist Tai Chi gave us health credits we could draw on for the future. It was a statement that stuck in my mind and really made sense.

It was less than two years ago that I had, once again, to take up the challenge of a diagnosis of cancer, this time breast cancer. To say that I was devastated is an understatement. It has been from that time till the present that I have really understood what Tai Chi has done for me in my life.

I was in a situation in my life where I had to made big decisions about treatment and very major surgery. But I was grateful early diagnosis had, once again, saved my life and decided whatever I had to do to keep myself going, well I would. The surgery I was to have meant I would have some major restrictions with movement of my arms and back which may be short term or permanent. In fact, I was told that I may not get my arms above my head ever again. Naturally my thoughts on what I would be able to do in my life, including my Tai Chi, were up there with all the other emotions and fears I was dealing with.

The rehabilitation exercises given to women with breast cancer are very limited and I can see why people do develop problems, especially with poor lymphatic drainage and restricted arm movement.

Well I could write a lot about my Tai Chi progress, especially over the first few weeks after surgery. But just to give you a brief rundown, when I left hospital two weeks after surgery I was doing most of the standing arm exercises. At each weekly visit my surgeon was constantly amazed at my mobility and speed of recovery. He kept asking me what I was doing and got me to show him the Tai Chi I was doing. *Those health credits were certainly evident.* It has taken me a good 18 months to be able to do the set without great back pain on completion, but everything seems to be functioning well and I am about to get my two year clearance from the specialist.

All I can say is that knowing Tai Chi gave me something constant to work with at a very bad time of my life. I know that without it and the kindness and love of my great family and wonderful friends I may not be as well and happy as I am today.

SEVEN

Chanting and Meditation

*T*HE CROSS-CULTURAL dialogue and exchange set up by Mr Moy, and continued by the International Taoist Tai Chi Society, to make the riches of traditional Chinese culture available to the West include the practices of chanting and meditation. They also include other Taoist arts, such as opening, closing and generally caring for the Taoist shrines at some Society sites and observing festivals associated with them. These practices are not empty or formulaic rituals, but physical and spiritual exercises that complement *Taoist Tai Chi*™ *taijiquan*. Just as they bring enormous benefits to people in all health conditions, so do chanting, meditation and the other Taoist temple arts. In fact, generally the people who have gained the most benefit from participating in the Society and its activities are those who practise both these arts and Taoist meditation and chanting. They are not esoteric practices, but physically and spiritually challenging and rewarding activities that re-align the body, relax body and mind, deepen breathing, resonate through the internal organs and energize every part of the body. They are vital for some people for recovering health and so are important components of health recovery stories.

Some people, who have already told their stories in previous chapters about learning or teaching *Taoist Tai Chi*™ *taijiquan* in an ordinary beginners' class, or in a Health Recovery class, or at a Health Recovery Program and about its effects on them, also have stories to tell about chanting and meditation and their effects on them. 'Have you done chanting and meditation?' became a standard question. It was not in the original schedule of standard questions (presented in the introduction), but it soon became a standard question, as chanting and meditation are integral and vital to the Health Recovery programs, and process, at the Orangeville Centre, and to the experience of health recovery and stories about it. At the Centre both were 'sold' on the basis of pain relief, re-alignment and relaxation for health recovery. This chapter explores chanting and meditation, their complementarity with other *Taoist Tai Chi*™ internal arts of health and their contribution to health recovery. Dee Steverson says:

> I do the chanting as much as I can because if I've had a sinus headache it won't get worse and it will go away. After doing Tai Chi for probably eight years, I found that the benefits I got from the Tai Chi were the same as I felt after the chanting, after the Lok Hup. They all had the same effect on my body and it was a very nice effect. So I don't separate them.

Lok Hup Ba Fa, to give it its full name, is a set of moves like Tai Chi that Mr Moy taught. He also founded the Gei Pang Lok Hup Academy to preserve and transmit this art. It is older than *taijiquan* and is considered more of an 'internal art.' In order to try to avoid any elitism associated with Lok Hup, Mr Moy said that everything you need for health is in *Taoist Tai Chi*™ *taijiquan* and that Lok Hup is an accelerator for your development. Most people who learn this art do so after practising *taijiquan* for a year or two at least.

Finding that stillness

The training in Taoism and *taijiquan* is not just physical and physiological, but also holistic and spiritual. Moreover, the physical and physiological are not confined to *taijiquan*, nor the holistic and spiritual to chanting and meditation. *Taoist Tai Chi*™ *taijiquan* is holistic and spiritual (and physical and physiological), and chanting and meditation are physical and physiological (and holistic and spiritual). Nor are all of these confined outside everyday life in some special space or place, but can, and should be, an integral part of everyday life. Chanting and

meditation are seemingly activities that you do outside the round of
activities and stress associated with everyday life, such as a job or a
family. The challenge is to take the calm and relaxed state produced by
both into everyday life, and sustain it there. Kelly Ekman says:

> I started to think about the physiology because in those days
> one of the medical advisers to the Society had started to come
> out to British Columbia and had started to do some physiology
> workshops. I started to come back to the Centre at Orangeville
> and come to the various workshops that were here. The more I
> came, the more I became involved and intrigued and started to
> look at it on a different level. It was kind of neat actually working
> on my stuff and working on everyone else's stuff. Lots of personal
> changes. Tai Chi is not just about the physical; it's a whole person
> experience. It was definitely a physiological experience, but it was
> as much an emotional and spiritual transformation as ever.
>
> There was a point when I was profoundly interested in learning
> about meditation and finding that stillness because there is a part
> of me that has the capacity to be incredibly still. I have always
> had that capacity but it seems to happen when I take myself out
> of activities, when no motion is required. When I am not busy
> I have the capacity for total stillness and I enjoy that, but what
> I was trying to find was how to take that stillness from those
> quiet moments and take it into those extremely busy moments,
> because the reality and nature of my life is that I always seem to
> be in a really high-stress or busy or complex environment. It's easy
> to be still when you absent yourself from the world, but it's much
> more difficult to be still when you're in a world that's incredibly
> challenging. By nature, my mind moves at speed all the time. I'm
> always multi-thinking, always multi-tasking. To be able to do that
> and to be calm at the same time – because I wasn't quite willing to
> give up that – and I haven't got it yet, of course, I haven't got that
> quality. I have tastes of it; I have moments when I can do it, but it's
> quite a ways to go. At least I know what I'm going for. So that's a
> huge part of what the Society offers. It's just a huge part.

Feeling something

Meditation, like *Taoist Tai Chi™ taijiquan*, is a means to an end, not an end in itself. They are both part of the same package of recovering physical, spiritual and mental health and well-being. They are integral facets of the International Taoist Tai Chi Society whose whole is more than the sum of its parts: *Taoist Tai Chi™ taijiquan*, Lok Hup, chanting, meditation, festivals, opening and closing shrines, organizing banquets and other events, running fundraising activities, being social and so on. David Kroh says:

I've definitely started doing some chanting and a little bit of meditation. I'd like to do a lot more but in terms of accreditation, there's nobody in our particular club who's accredited to teach it. Whatever opportunities come up that I can possibly make, I make. The chanting is really wonderful. A long time ago, many moons ago, I used to be in a choir at the church that I attended. I can remember feeling something back then. I didn't really know what it was and it was after a lot of singing. This is a little bit different. It's a lot more; it's a lot more deep; it's a lot more powerful; it's a lot more fast-acting; it starts happening much sooner. It opens everything up in the chest region, in the neck and in the face. It's easier to breathe; it's easier to relax.

I find after chanting that it's getting back that similar meditative quality that Tai Chi has. So you don't necessarily have to do the Tai Chi but you can also do the chanting and you can get some similar kinds of things going on. This past Health Recovery week was a wonderful experience for me in the sense that I had done some chanting earlier and then, in the evening, we did some meditation. I could still hear the chanting going on in my head, or whatever you want to call it. I could still experience the chanting going on while I was meditating which again was something very relaxing and calming.

I've got tons and tons to learn and experience. As much as I delve into this it never ceases to amaze me how much more there is. It's kind of like climbing a mountain with the whole range

in front of me. There are times, once in a while, when no matter
how much you work, you're not necessarily going to get there, but
what does that mean? In the overall scheme of things I look at it
like this: if it was easy and there was no challenge to it, it would be
boring and there would be a block. There's lots to it; it's exciting;
there's never an end and that's good. It keeps you going.

Get rid of the noise

David has been an Assistant at a Health Recovery Program and
experienced a lot of benefits from chanting and meditation. What about
the participants, who usually have serious health conditions? What is
their experience of chanting and meditation? Have they experienced
any benefits? Is chanting and meditation for them too? Andy Ferenc
has MS and uses a walking frame to get around. He usually shuffles
around, dragging one leg after the other, using his walking frame for
support. One night after meditating he was using the parallel bars to
hold on to and he was jumping off the floor. He says:

> I've done meditation before, but I wasn't really conscious of
> what I should expect from it. I thought I'm just going to sit there
> and get rid of the noise in my head that seems to rattle through
> there all the time like electricity. There's always something in there
> that always seems to keep the brain rattling. I never really thought
> about it until this year. There had been various situations that I had
> had. For instance, the first one started off with one Instructor. This
> was the first session that we had of meditation and, again, I wasn't
> too sure what I was supposed to expect for myself. The next stage
> was with another Instructor and there was a little bit more that
> was clicking with me but, again, I wasn't confident in myself about
> what it was I was going to achieve with it. Then with yet another
> Instructor he did a little more, and then I started to understand a
> little bit more about what I should expect of myself.
>
> During this Health Recovery week we are starting to do more
> meditation. It's all just started to come together, especially in the
> last week when a different Instructor altogether was leading the

meditation session. We were sitting meditating and then all of a sudden there was something inside that kind of clicked in me and I felt more comfortable. I felt more relaxed and some of the noise in the head went away. I'm not saying that I'm mentally retarded or anything. It's just that some of the chitchat that goes on had gone. It just felt better; it felt stronger. I got up that first evening and I approached an Assistant and asked him if he would help me do the snakes. The snakes were powerful that particular evening and I did the jumping that gave me that spring. The walking was unbelievable. I thought at the time that I must have either relaxed in my body, or the stress factor may have been gone, or that there was more of a positive energy inside my body. I just felt at that moment, when I got up and asked if he would help me, that it just all came together. It only lasted a short time, but boy it was pretty dynamic for me.

There was another situation I had a number of months ago with one of the Instructors who was doing a lot of work with me at the time. He took me aside on the third day and he really fine-tuned the Dan Yus that I was doing – freestanding. I thought that was kind of strange, but I decided to go with the flow. Every time I did it there was a minor adjustment that he would do for me. I don't know how many times we had done it and then there was a point where he said, 'Sit and relax'. I said, 'No, no, just let me do a couple more'. He did a couple more adjustments, and with the final adjustment, there was something that opened up inside me. Everything just started to flow, energy, blood, I don't know what it was. I fell down in my chair. I couldn't even stand on my feet anymore. I started to cry like I've never cried before. I don't mind admitting that. It was an incredible feeling inside, a warm rush of energy that was a vibration in the legs and the back. I couldn't even control myself. I had no clue about what was going on and I couldn't walk.

It was lunchtime and the bell had rung and I asked everyone to just leave me there. I just want to think about what just went through me. I had my cane with me, as the Instructor had said,

'You're going to be walking so you had better go get your cane before we do anything'. Then about half an hour or so later I got up and sat on the floor and started to meditate for a while, just to try and absorb everything that had happened to me. Then I got my cane and walked down the hall and around the washroom and back into the hall. An Assistant came in and saw me walking and said, 'What's going on?' I said. 'I don't know, I just had to walk.' That was the first of two events.

The second event happened the same night. It was around 2.30. Something told me to wake up. I woke up and something again said, 'Get up and walk.' I got up. I took my cane without putting it on the ground. I just held it in my hand and I walked down to the hall in the dark. There were a few people in there doing their set. I started to yell and scream and I said, 'You've got to see this; you've got to see this! It's unbelievable. You guys put in all this work. You've got to see what happens.' I walked around the hall twice without the cane touching the ground, came down the stairs, had a little snack, came back up the stairs, walked around the hall one more time, down the passage back to my room and I went back to sleep again. It was just spectacular. I thought, 'Oh, my God! What an incredible breakthrough.' It may not happen again. Who knows?

At least I know what that experience was all about. Maybe if I work hard enough, maybe it will come back again. It was incredible. I just enjoyed it so much. I had asked a senior Instructor, who had worked closely with Master Moy, if anything like this had happened to him. He said that he had once had a similar experience with Master Moy who had helped him. He looked at me and it took him back as well to what he had gone through. Then he didn't talk about it too much so I didn't pursue it. I know he's a very private man. He doesn't like to talk about his achievements or about helping others.

Chanting and meditation can, and do, have wonderful effects and enormous benefits. Other activities, and even the ambience of the Centre at Orangeville, have calming effects. The property has a Taoist shrine housed in a converted old barn away from the main building and nestled beneath maple trees. This was a favourite place of mine during my stay there. It is a focus and venue for chanting and meditation with its pictures and kneeling stools. I would go and chant with others during organized sessions, or go by myself to meditate at every opportunity at other times in the afternoon, or in evening before going to bed after a full day of *taijiquan*. It is a place of quietness and stillness in the middle of the activity and noise of the programs and workshops at the Centre.

The shrine is calming

The Centre is staffed and run largely by volunteers who come for several weeks or months to help run the place. People who come for programs and workshops also help to run the place by doing the daily chores. The volunteers often play the role of information-providers about how the place is run, what to do and where supplies are stored, or trainers in how to use the equipment. They also tend to go around doing the jobs, or finishing the jobs the people on the programs or workshops don't do, or don't finish. One of them cares for the shrine. Micheline Blaquière had been a volunteer for many months. Caring for the shrine for her was not a burdensome chore, but a calming practice. She says:

> Staying here, I have had a lot of help from many persons, particularly the Health Recovery weeks for my physical part. Kelly helped me a lot with the mental part because I was very overactive. Very much. To me, she was a little bit like me. She explained to me how to calm down, so that was a big gift because everybody was always telling me, 'Calm down, calm down', since I was 4 years old, but nobody taught me how. She took like 15 minutes to explain that to me, and it works. I increased my sleep hours from 4 hours to 6 hours about 2 weeks after that. At a Health Recovery week the teacher started to work with me on my neck. Something was wrong with my neck position. For 2 days now, I catch 8 hours sleep. Easy. I don't know, but there's something there.

Kelly told me the first thing to do to calm down was to contemplate nature. Look at nature. Two minutes is enough, I told her. No, she said, you have to sit and watch, look at the trees, look at the things closely, take the time to look at each part of the tree, and so that helped me a lot to take a walk each day. She told me to increase my meditation. I was going one time a day. She told me two times, so I did. She gave me the responsibility of the shrine. That started me slowly in the morning and it slowed my pace at night. I think that helps with my sleeping also. I think it's that.

The shrine is calming me down because in the shrine, with the rituals, personally, if I have to do it, I do it well. Kelly and others explained to me that you must move slowly in the shrine. Use delicate things to work in the shrine. I don't carry the big pot of oil. I have a bottle of oil to fill the lamps and, when there's no more oil, come back slowly and fill the bottle again, and go back. So that was pacing me down. Doing the salutations when offering the incense sticks also helps to calm me down because to start the day it warms up that part of your spine and it takes the stress out of the back.

The atmosphere is very calm in there, and peaceful. It's under trees. You don't hear the noise as much as in the Health Recovery building so it's calming you down. You have to walk along up to there. If someone is with you, you have to say, 'I'm sorry, I have to go and do the shrine.' You walk along and that starts already the process of calming down.

I had a big experience with chanting, chanting and Tai Chi. I was chanting in Health Recovery weeks, sometimes in the shrine, but that week, we did chanting very early in the morning, up in the hall, doing Tai Chi right after it, like just walking back to the hall and doing Tai Chi. I realized, coming to the third part of the Tai Chi, set my energy was circulating so fast. The first time I had what I thought was Angina, but it was not Angina so the Instructor put me on the bars doing Dan Yus to regulate the circulation. I did not know what was happening to me, but I decided to trust them and do what they told me. I did Dan Yus at the bar, about 100 of them. It came back.

The day after I met Kelly and she told me to try doing Tai Chi after chanting for one day so everything was all right. The day after I tried chanting again and during Tai Chi the reaction was the same, but there was more circulation of I don't know what. It went up the back and this time it stopped between the shoulder blades. I had in the back the same kind of reaction as I had in the front two days before. I went by myself to the bar to do Dan Yus, but after doing them I had to rest. I had to go and rest for an hour. The next day I tried chanting without Tai Chi and it was fine.

The day after I tried chanting and Tai Chi and then everything flowed very easily. No more pain and a very good feeling of – I don't know how you say that – it was circulating more, but very regular and agreeable. Since then I do a lot of chanting, like I did in Fung Loy Kok week. We did a chant that is eighteen pages long. After the first eight pages my eyes started to drip and something else was coming out from under the external part of the eye. I was yawning and yawning. I had to stop chanting after eight pages. The day after I could go up to twelve pages. The day after I did eighteen pages before it started dripping. There's something, I don't know what, in there.

Fung Loy Kok week is a training program in the Taoist temple arts and in chanting and meditation. Mr Moy co-founded the Fung Loy Kok Institute of Taoism to promote the translation and study of the Taoist texts as well as training in the temple arts. The Institute is a registered charitable organization in Canada and is a focus for the philanthropic, community-service work of the International Taoist Tai Society.

I have a little form of asthma, and the chanting improves the air. It's easy for me to know because usually I cannot go where there are cleaning products, like in the cleaning supply room. I was not able to go there when I first came here. My air tube was sticking together and I couldn't breathe anymore. Now I can go there and fill a bucket of water and go out – no problem. I can go in the space where they wash dishes and use cleaning products and I'm okay. But there are some I cannot breathe close to still. I can tolerate dishwashing, cleaning products and Windex, but Shockwave is pretty hard for me. I feel sick but maybe I'll get used to this one too.

Train for life and death

Micheline has had a lot of benefits from chanting that are both physiological and psychological. Besides being physiological and psychological, chanting is also spiritual, as Kelly has suggested. It connects with the spirit world within us and around us. Naturally some people have difficulty in accepting the existence of such a world or in coming to terms with how to relate to it. Other people come to terms with it, though they may not feel comfortable with it. One such person is Peter Turner who says:

> During the week of the anniversary of the D'Arcy Street Temple in Toronto, chanters from Hong Kong were here at Orangeville. They came and spent a week at the Centre and they chanted every morning and every evening and purified the place for us. They just transformed the spirit of this place during that week. I was fortunate enough to be here, call it a coincidence, but I do not really believe in that concept any more. They were chanting all the time and I was planting rose beds.
>
> One of the things that happened during that period was that the meteorological phenomena, which occur when chanting takes place, were experienced directly, not just heard about in stories. This place had been in drought for six weeks. Everywhere around had rain but this place had had nothing. The chanters come, and absolutely to order the heavens open. I spent quite a lot of time swabbing out the hall during these tremendous storms, and lightning comes down, and wind splits the tree next to where I am working. This was just amazing, but it was always in time with the chanting, so much so, and you would say that, having studied climatology, meteorology would give me some idea of how these things work. Most of this stuff may be coincidence, but it was a different kind of experience and linkage to a different set of possibilities.

I had always been fearful of the spiritual side of this tradition. I had dabbled in thought-transference and meditation and stuff. I had a couple of scary experiences, so I kind of had this door open and left some stuff behind it. I've tried to park it for about the last ten years, so I guess basically not being able to open up into that area was hard for me. The only part of the whole process that was shut down for me was this area that I did not like to go into, in my dreams more than anything else. During that week that was transformed as the chanters were very keen to explain everything. For them the spirit and the body world were the same.

On one day, for example, there were three characters, restless spirits, who came into the entrance hall here while they were chanting. The chanters changed the chant, a four-hour chant, they all saw them and they all changed the chant because they weren't able to appease them, basically telling them to stay away from this place of healing. So this is just straight dialogue between the chanters themselves. I am giving a context for why for me there was something much more profound here than just the physiological.

I remember the first time Master Moy said that meditation was a preparation for death in a series of sessions that went from five minutes to forty minutes of pain. So after that experience, just before he died, I was more comfortable with this, whereas until a few weeks before that, it was parked in this area I didn't want to go. I am not looking to take anybody there, but to be comfortable being there, to be able to be there for someone who has not accepted it, and is facing it. We focused in the Health Recovery Instructor week, for example, on an interview with an erudite scholar who had just found out he was dying of cancer. For about an hour, we just listened, to help people realise that this is where we are all going. In health recovery we are dealing with this; in long term care we are dealing with this; everybody we meet will have to deal with this: just caring for folk transitioning out of the world and seeing how these take expression in three areas: health recovery, quiet cultivation and long-term care. In the first instance, for example, we might just focus on the health benefits of chanting.

It's the same for meditation, the process is more like having a quiet conversation with a good friend, a gentle process of relaxation. An approach to the whole person, so whether in classes, specifically health recovery, trying to find out where somebody is in their lives, what stage they are at in their lives, so if somebody has an emotional response the instinct is sometimes to go in close to support them. This instinct is not always best, it's just what they are going through. If somebody is going up and down doing rows of brush knees, bawling their eyes out, that's fine. If somebody who was doing a standing exercise and collapsed on the floor, Master Moy would walk away, when everyone was crowding around. 'Why don't you listen to your body, why did you wait till it falls over, it's your responsibility.'

So an understanding of personal responsibility comes in all of this. For some, the challenge may be appropriate: so, for example, if they are paraplegic, walking up and down stairs may be where they want to be, others may want to walk in the park. We need to be sensitive too, if their spirit is driving them beyond where their body can go, to be able to be there before they fall over and damage themselves, and that's important because they could set themselves back for months. For example, somebody walking using the parallel bars, if you're not there at the very moment they collapse, they can end up with broken legs. It's about trying to find a balance between the reality of what their body can do and our understanding.

So I really want to understand how the body works, become more aware of the power of the conversation with the spirit, understanding what makes somebody tick, and the ability of people to progress their Tai Chi – their development is more in this area. So in a class or a workshop, it may not be the physical correction that has the greatest impact on them. So it is about creating a better environment to help people train for life and death, for example, in Health Recovery when somebody with a frozen shoulder is put in a group with people with coronary bypasses or cancer, that preoccupation with themselves dissolves. Initially they see themselves and focus on that, until they realise there is a range of challenges that people have. This is the importance of the oral tradition, as this is very hard to achieve in an hour-and-a-half class. People come for a variety of reasons, but they stay because of the transformational experience which they value, be it emotional, spiritual or physical, and appreciating the linkage between those.

So we have the propriety and richness of this tradition, the rigorous discipline, but with my interest in the martial and the monastic, an almost acolyte-type intensity was my propensity. Now I am much softer. Sometimes it is like triage. If someone wants to cry all over you, it's okay. If the next person's problem is their ego, and the person in the next room needs physical help, quiet helps you to be where you need to be. To be asked to balance up the needs and the energy of the folk, such as this week where we have sixty people, more than thirty of whom are Participants, most of the Assistants coming with baggage, we need to create an environment in which that can dissolve, which happens once you get the chemistry right, juxtaposition of Participants and Assistants.

I remember last year at Continuing Instructor-in-Training week, an Instructor from Australia led with a very different style. He just did the move about thirty times and said nothing. Later he shared that Master Moy had said, 'don't talk about the internals, just trust in the form and the healing will come.' So for me this has a resonance of expression, because if I hadn't had the accidents I would probably have been even more intense. I am quieter now and the depth of conviction just increases. Reading this you probably think the intensity is still pretty strong. I am very aware of the gift, of the rich tradition we have to explore and to share. And for those that come to Taoist Tai Chi with a little understanding, that it takes patience to create the opportunities for sharing, the Society is inherently inefficient, but it's part of its nature, and it's very good. Most important is the way we do things.

The Society has two levels of instructors: beginner instructors and continuing instructors-in-training. The Society offers training programs for both levels. After beginners have learnt the basic moves of the *Taoist Tai Chi*™ *taijiquan* 'set' they can go on into a continuing class with a continuing instructor-in-training to refine and develop this art and to learn and practise other arts such as Dan Yus, Tor Yus and snakes.

Master Moy has cropped up as a topic of conversation time and again in this and previous chapters as having said this or done that. He has also figured prominently as a leading character in many people's stories about their experience of learning the *Taoist Tai Chi*™ internal arts of health. This is understandable as he was the teacher and source of these arts, and the founder of the International Taoist Tai Chi Society. He is the pivot or axis around which all its activities and practices revolved and evolved, and continue to revolve and evolve. It is time to acknowledge and explore his pivotal role so he is the topic of the next chapter.

EIGHT

Master Moy

NO BOOK about the *Taoist Tai Chi*™ internal arts of health that retells some of its health recovery stories, and especially the first book about it intended for a general readership (as distinct from its own self-published instruction guides and manuals and translations of Taoist texts intended for its members and practitioners) would be complete without an account of, or a chapter about, its founder, Master Moy Lin-Shin (1931-1998). Perhaps appropriately it is the longest chapter in this book, though there is much more that could be said. The inclusion of such a chapter is not done out of any sense of merely fulfilling an obligation to his memory, or the desire to indulge in hero-worship, or to write a 'saint's story' (hagiography). Nor is the dedication of this book to his memory just a ritualistic or polite gesture, the done thing. Just as chanting and meditation became natural topics of conversation in the interviews I conducted as the basis for this book so did the question, 'did you ever meet Mr Moy?'

My aim in asking the question was to gain, and gather together, some impressions about him, to gauge the effect he had on other's lives even if they had not met him, and to preserve both, not only for posterity but also for the present. The aim was not to research a biography, or even to collect anecdotes about him, though there are quite a few of them in what follows. Again, these are only the tip of an iceberg. These have now passed into the Society, and are passed on in it, as what one member calls 'Mr Moyisms.' 'Mr Moy said this,' 'Mr Moy said that.'

There is definitely a desire here to respect his memory, to express gratitude for the gifts he gave and to pass on his oral teaching, especially to those who never met him, but there is also a danger in invoking his name simply as an authority to arbitrate debates. He certainly taught, and expected, obedience and respect, but he also taught principles and virtues, and expected enterprise and initiative. Finding the balance here is a lifelong task. He disliked people waiting for him to tell them what to do. And there is plenty of that to be going on with in following the aims and objectives of the Society.

My aim in asking the question 'did you ever meet Mr Moy?' was, and in including this chapter is, to acknowledge his role in founding the International Taoist Tai Chi Society and in teaching the *Taoist Tai Chi™* internal arts of health and passing on their health benefits, to allow others the opportunity to express their gratitude and respect for his having done so (as the dedication does on my part too), to record their experience of meeting him (or not) and the impression he made on them, and so to tell their story about the part he played explicitly or implicitly in their health recovery story. He has figured already as a leading actor in many of the health recovery stories presented in this book. In this chapter he figures not so much as an instructor of *Taoist Tai Chi™ taijiquan*, of how to do a move or as a source of techniques, but as a teacher of Taoism, of how to be more compassionate, how to look after other people, how to be a better person, how to be more centred, but less self-centred. These lessons are probably harder to learn than those about how to do a move or perform a sequence.

Although this chapter focuses on Mr Moy, it is not a biography. I think he would be appalled if anyone were to write a biography of him, though there is certainly plenty of material out there besides the anecdotes about him that circulate in the Society and the brief biography of him on the Society website in the page headed 'Our Founder.' His older sister, Mrs Lee, is in her 80s and lives in New York. She has many interesting stories to tell about him and I heard some of them when she visited the Orangeville centre to pay her annual respects to her brother whose ashes are interred in the Columbarium there (see the frontispiece to this book). If I had wanted to write a biography of him,

I would have interviewed her. It would go against a basic Taoist virtue of egolessness though. He certainly was a very remarkable man as this chapter (if not all the preceding ones) testify, but he was a self-effacing, yet strong-willed, person who lived an austere, yet rich, and rewarding life. He was multifaceted and paradoxical, yet simple, and so on. His vision and legacy are amazing.

The experience of meeting him changed some people's lives forever. Some people were only with him for three hours, some for many years. Both had profound, life-changing experiences. Some people did not meet him, but still feel that they know him. One such person is Raymonde Southey from Montreal who says:

> I started classes in the fall of '97. He passed away in June '98. This coincided with a National Workshop that was supposed to be Master Moy's. When we got there we learnt that he had just passed away the night before. A senior Instructor gave the workshop. We did a lot of meditation that day. It was difficult for those who had known him. It was expected, but still… Even though I didn't meet him, I've heard so much about him that I feel that I know him. I would describe him as a humble, very kind person with an extraordinary vision of what the International Taoist Tai Chi Society should be. Selfless. Just wanting to help people. He must have been extremely intelligent to have a vision like that. It's just amazing, starting from nothing. A little club and then travelling back and forward from Toronto to Montreal after his work. This is how it started. It's amazing. It's an example. A lot of senior people in the Society have tried to bring that out and tell us about it.

Like Raymonde, Micheline Blaquière did not meet him, but says:

> I miss him. I miss him because I'm kind of bad news for some teachers who ask me what I would have done if Mr Moy had been there. If Mr Moy had been there, I would have followed him like a tu-tu. A tu-tu is a little dog in French who follows. They say, 'You don't follow easily. Why not?' 'Because you're not Mr Moy!' There's a difference. The difference is that I know that they learnt from him. I know that they want to give, but they do not have the experience he had. They do not have all the knowledge that he

had. He has all of it; they have part of it. I never know if I can trust the little part that they have. That is why I am kind of missing him, but I manage.

I see what they are doing with somebody else, when I see that they are helping somebody else. Like I saw Andy Ferenc doing his 60 Dan Yus and he cannot do it without collapsing with his knees 20 minutes before. A senior Instructor who was a student of Mr Moy comes here and finds a way to align him correctly and stays beside him keeping him aligned and then that guy does 60 good Dan Yus. Now you cannot question that. An Instructor from Montreal realized I had hurt my hip. He gave me a way to do my Tor Yus to prevent that. Then you realize that some of them know a lot. You come to recognise them, the way they look at you. You kind of realize that you can trust them. It's not the way they do their Tai Chi. It's the way they look and the way they help you.

I don't know what they see, but they see something. Like with Andy and his instructor who said to me, 'Go and get his cane. He doesn't need his walker to walk. He can walk.' I went and got his cane. I was an Assistant that week. We looked at him walk and he didn't use the cane to walk. He used the cane to recover his balance. He's out of balance. Then we started to count the number of steps he took before he lost his balance. There were four, five steps, and sometimes six, and sometimes three, but he was able to walk without his cane. We decided that if he can walk three steps without his cane, he can do Dan Yus. We put a special set-up for him so he could recover his balance if something happened. The set-up we did was very simple. We put a chair next to the parallel bar so that if he lost his balance he could put his elbow on the bar to recover his balance. With the chair and the bar he had a lot of confidence. He did sixty very nice Dan Yus. Wow!

A good spiritual director

Besides the people who did not meet Mr Moy, but were still affected by him, are the tens of thousands of people who did meet him and were affected by him too. He had a remarkable capacity to remember people from many different countries around the world after just a couple of meetings. One person who did meet him and for whom he always had a smile was Helen Christian who said:

The thing I observe – I'm a psychologist by training – I observe people and I like doing that, it's almost automatic – it's so fascinating to observe how people relate even to the memory of Master Moy. I've learned more about him since he died than when he was alive because people tell stories about him, the way they do about people who have died. He strikes me, listening to people talk about him, as what we would call a good spiritual director. He seems to know what to say to people to really strike them, what's good for them. I greatly admire that trait. It's hard for me to tolerate some of the almost worship. I never got the feeling that he was asking for it. I met him several times. I never got the feeling that he was asking people to kow-tow and bow down and call him 'master.' I've been struck time and time again by his common sense. He was a really sensible guy. Some people practically pray to him. I felt that he didn't *ask* for it. Some people think I'm wrong about that. I don't know what those other individual things are because I was missing something. I never thought he was asking to be sifu, or a guru. What was he like? I said that he was a terrific spiritual director, but I never knew him well enough to have that kind of relationship with him at all. An immensely practical man. Talented. Look at what he did! Pretty amazing.

The legacy he left includes the International Taoist Tai Chi Centre at Orangeville, centres around the world, the idea for the construction of the long-term care facility, and an international Society active in 28 countries around the world. Basically one man achieved all that in 28 years – one country per year on average.

Helen has raised an important topic of debate about what Mr or Master Moy saw himself as, what he wanted to be called and whether he should be referred to as 'Mister' or 'Master'. This topic has been lurking in the background of the two previous storytellers' accounts of *not* meeting him. Raymonde referred to him as 'Master,' Micheline as 'Mr.'

My usage has varied too. I addressed him as 'Mr' and referred to him as such when he was alive and when I conducted the interviews for this book. However, I have entitled this chapter 'Master Moy' as this book is addressed to the general public and intended for the general reader. Dr Peter Cook, the Executive Director of the Taoist Tai Chi Society of Australia, traces the lineage and nuances of these different usages, and the different occasions and contexts in which it is appropriate to use which title:

When I lived in Canada in the 80s, my recollection is that virtually everyone called Mr Moy 'Mr'. 'Master' was used only for more formal purposes, and perhaps when speaking to members of the public. There is a certain element here of wanting to convey Mr Moy's stature to the public – that is, he is/was a Master. But for internal purposes, most people for some reason were more comfortable with Mr. I did hear from someone that, initially at least, Mr Moy did not want to be called 'Sifu', which is the Chinese equivalent of Master (my understanding is that this term means 'respected teacher'). There were some ways in which Mr Moy did not want all the formal trappings of his status. Hence, perhaps, the use of 'Mr' by us English speakers conveys the right combination of respect and informality that Mr Moy seemed to like. Nevertheless, it is said that his followers in the Chinese community in Toronto called him Sifu anyway (as did I sometimes when I greeted him). I notice that in recent times, there seems to be a greater use of the term 'Master' when referring to Mr Moy. I speculate that one reason for this is that an increasing proportion of (newer) members of the Society either did not meet Mr Moy, or met him only rarely. Therefore there is more a feeling of the need to refer to his formal status.

Understanding and observing the protocol is part of the training in Taoism. Heath Greville, a Director of the International Taoist Tai Chi Society, sums up the situation succinctly:

Some people accepted Mr Moy as their Master and referred to him as 'Master.' Some called him 'Mr' and accepted him as Master. Some called him 'Mr' and accepted him as a teacher. That's my understanding of some of the reasons for the differing usage of the titles. As far as I know, he never asked or expected anyone to call him Master.

I have let the varied usages of the interviewees stand for these reasons as they convey some of this variety of people's relationships with him. He did not, however, as Judy Millen puts it, 'form personal attachments' with his students. He had what Kelly Ekman calls 'a calm detachment' which some people took as coldness or aloofness. Some people who attended his workshops expected him to perform for them. He refused to fulfil this expectation. He would bring with him instructors who he was training to lead workshops. He would sit in the background and just when you thought he was asleep he would say something like 'timing,' or 'drop elbows,' or 'stretch.' He was usually more alert and observant than most people gave him credit for. Yet he certainly did not adopt the position of the all-seeing, all-knowing master onto whom the student transferred their desires and fears. Someone who washes out his Y-front underpants by hand and hangs them out publicly on a chair to dry in the sun is hardly your archetypal master!

The softest hand

Some people had some remarkable experiences when they met him, especially, and initially, if they shook his hand. His handshake was famous, so famous in fact that some people shook his hand just to experience it – at first-hand as it were! He probably got sick of that, though usually he was very generous with his time and energy. Dee Steverson said that when she met Mr Moy, he told her she should practise the *Taoist Tai Chi*™ internal arts of health twenty-four hours a day, not in the sense of doing the moves or exercises all day and night, but in the sense of being aligned and calm, and performing the physical activities of everyday life in accordance with its 'bio-mechanically sound' and spiritually centred principles. She says:

> The first time I met him I was totally amazed. I shook his hand. His hand was the softest hand I have ever touched in my life. He only gave me one correction one time. He noticed that my circulation

was very bad. I had very bad circulation where my lips were blue when I started Tai Chi. They're no longer blue, but I'm still very poorly circulated. Through an interpreter he told me that I needed to take Chinese herbs. I asked him which ones. He couldn't explain it or he knew that I would not be able to get them in Tallahassee. So he told the interpreter for me to buy beef and cook the beef in a broth and drink the beef broth. And that was his correction. I did it for a short while. It's not my favourite thing.

What really helped with my blue lips is that I would do brush knees every day. Before I would go to work I would do at least a hundred of them. And within a month or two the blue lips went away. I have to do it every day. At one of the workshops Master Moy said do Tai Chi twenty-four hours a day. I really got turned on to that idea. So I find in all different kinds of ways that you can do Tai Chi. I'll talk to people and it never occurs to them that vacuuming a floor is a Tor Yu, that when you have to look under the sink to find something, you Dan Yu down. Opening a heavy door is a Tor Yu. So it's fun to find ways that you can put Tai Chi into your everyday life. When you really get your spine nice and loose to sweep it is so easy.

What's he doing?

Besides meeting him and getting dietary, medicinal or other practical advice then and there, other people attended workshops with him and had remarkable experiences with him there. Some people, like Bill Robichaud, went to a workshop with Mr Moy very early on in their journey. In a previous chapter Bill said that initially his training in anatomy and physiology was a hindrance to his understanding of the *Taoist Tai Chi*™ internal arts of health. When he attended his first workshop with Mr Moy and saw what he did, he was unable to compute these arts in terms of anatomy and physiology. Bill says he met Mr Moy on two occasions:

The first time I think I had just finished my first beginner class and he was coming to Tallahassee for a Tai Chi week. I was all excited.

I thought, 'Gee, I can't even do a set. Even if I'm in the middle of a group, I'll probably stumble over my feet. I can't remember any of this but, boy, if I go to that Tai Chi week with Master Moy, I can come out of there, I can do it.' I was all excited I was going to go to Tallahassee and I made arrangements for that and met Master Moy there. Unfortunately after the first day or at the end of the first day – of course, everyone there had been doing Tai Chi for a long time – so he said 'How would you like to learn Lok Hup? I'm looking around and asking people 'What's a low cup?' So that's what we did that week and it just screwed me up for about a good year. I mean, I didn't know Tai Chi and now I'm doing this and it was like I got it all mixed and I couldn't remember anything, but the experience of the meeting was somewhat at a distance like it wasn't like I would sit down and talk with him. Certainly watching what was going on and watching him work with someone.

A young man came in who had Leukaemia and I watched Master Moy work on him and saw a few things that really stopped me. I couldn't understand; I couldn't explain. Some of the things that were happening didn't make sense to me from my understanding of the body. The young man was sitting in the chair. He had come in using crutches because the Leukaemia was deteriorating his body enough to where his hips were a problem and his knees were a problem. He was about the colour of a sheet of writing paper. He was white. Leukaemia does that. Your circulation is really lousy. You're also anaemic and so you just lose all colour. So I was watching. He was in the chair and Master Moy was working on him and bending him back and forth and I don't know about the particulars watching from a distance what was he doing and the next thing he's smacking him a few times on the back and I thought, 'Gees, what's he doing? Poor guy comes in and he's got Leukaemia and now he's getting beat up. What's going on?' I knew he was helping him, but I just didn't understand how or what it was that he was doing.

And then I noticed, even from a pretty good distance, the young man started to get pink all over his body, he was getting colour and his skin was starting to get that glow you get when you first start to sweat a little bit. I thought, 'He's getting heated up. He's not doing it himself. Master Moy is doing something to him but his circulation is tremendously increased and he's heating up and his blood vessels are dilating and his skin is getting pinker as a result and he is trying to get rid of some excess heat. And it's like he's not even moving. Master Moy had to be doing something, he had to be putting energy into him somehow, but you can't do that.' It was just really amazing. I had no idea what was going on.

The second time I met him was when I was visiting in Toronto with some students. I was a director of a regional science fair and they had an international science fair outside of Toronto in one of the smaller cities with a university nearby. I thought, 'Well, while I'm here I need to rent a car and go into Toronto and see if I can find these places that I'd heard about and go to Bathurst St and D'Arcy St and see if I can find Master Moy and drop in and pay my respects.' That seemed to be a proper thing to do. So I eventually found my way to Toronto and wandered around for a while and found Bathurst and walked upstairs. I'd worn my Florida Tai Chi tee shirt so I would have some kind of recognition. I walked in and the next thing I know I'm being escorted over to sit down, and they're bringing me tea and they're bringing me cookies to eat and all this kind of neat stuff, and it's like they didn't know I was coming. I just walked in off the street and they're treating me like a long lost friend. I met two Health Recovery Instructors. I had no idea who they were. I'm having this really tremendous experience meeting these terrific people.

Master Moy was sitting in the back and I needed to go over and say hello. I knew I couldn't carry on a conversation and yet I needed to say hello. So he was in the back at a table playing Mah Jong with his buddies so I walked to the back and introduced myself and said, 'I just wanted to come by and say hello. I come from Florida and I wanted to thank you for all the help you have given me.' He looks up and goes, 'Okay' and goes back to playing Mah Jong. I stood there and thought, 'Well, alright.' I had to talk to myself, 'Bill, what do you expect him to do? You walk in off the street. He's having fun with his friends.'That was my second meeting. It wasn't an instructional time, but it taught me something.

Looking so normal

Mister Moy was always teaching and his students were learning something, whether it was how to do the second half of Lok Hup, or how to fold tee shirts properly, or serve spring rolls quickly because people were hungry. Unlike Bill, Ankie Boumans had not even finished the beginners' course before she went to a workshop with Mr Moy. She says:

> I did not know the entire set. Once he has been in Holland. I thought, 'Alright. This is my chance. I'm going to see that man.' At first I didn't dare. I thought, 'I can't do the set. Can I go?' The Instructor I had said, 'Just stay behind. It's okay. Just follow. Just stay behind someone.' So I once saw him. My husband still laughs about it. I had to drive for two hours. That's a long distance for Holland because it's a small country. I saw him and I thought, 'What a normal looking man.' I kind of expected a big guru and he was looking so normal, but with a lot of power. He had such a power. The way he looked it was so powerful for me and only that gave energy. I did not understand what happened. I drove home and came home at two in the morning. My husband was already sleeping and I woke him up. I said, 'Alright, you've got to wake up! You've got to know what I saw today! It was great!' I was bouncing around. Then he said, 'I'm sleeping.' 'Not anymore! You have to know this.' Well, it stayed like that for two days.

A calm detachment

Kelly Ekman also started going to workshops very early on whenever Mr Moy came out to British Columbia and led workshops from which she learnt a lot about what she calls his 'calm detachment' and about thinking, or *not* thinking. Like Ankie, she says:

The first time I met Mr Moy for a workshop I had not yet finished the beginners set – I think I was about two months into it. That was the first workshop I took with Mr Moy and that was a totally intriguing experience because at first, of course, one has an idea and expectation of what it's all going to be about. Mr Moy's method of teaching of course was quite neutral and quite different so that was a learning experience in itself. You started to understand the culture of the Society and starting to understand the lineage and the tradition and how the tradition was taught. Mr Moy would often appear to many people to be stand-offish. There was just a kind of calm detachment. It wasn't that he didn't care. It was that he just had this level of calm that came from a different place. It took me years of study to absorb and get a better sense of that. That was fun.

Right at the beginning I had a lot of contact and got a lot of personal help from Mr Moy over the years. He worked with me quite extensively on many different levels. I think he knew what I needed when I did see him. The first couple of years I would go to workshops and he would just kind of look at me. I don't recall that he actually gave me a formal correction, but he would sort of look at me and say, 'Re-lax.' After a couple of workshops like that he would look at me very intensely and say, 'Think-ing.' But of course that made me go away and think more about what he meant by 'Thinking.' Should I be thinking more or should I be thinking less? I was never quite clear. It still took me quite a few years to figure that one out a little bit. So those were amazingly little contacts, but amazingly rich contacts. Of course, the more I did, the more hooked I got.

A body of people

Judy Millen started learning *Taoist Tai Chi*™ *taijiquan* in 1979 so of all the people who tell their stories in this book she has been practising it the longest. She did a lot of work with Mr Moy from whom she learnt some valuable lessons, not so much in how to do a move, but in how to be a better, more compassionate and caring, person. Like a number of people, she had a very emotional response to something he said to her on one occasion. Part of the process of emotional healing can be crying and being upset. At other times, weeping tears of joy are part of the process. Being emotional, and dealing with it, can be part of the training for some people. This can occur not only when someone says something, but also when talking about the International Taoist Tai Chi Society, or practising *taijiquan*, or chanting, or meditating. Emotion is a part of life and emotional health is a part of being healthy. Although Taoism teaches that one should not be ruled by destructive or negative emotions, they need to be dealt with, calmed and transformed into creative and positive energy. Mr Moy was very sensitive to what people were feeling, to 'the emotional tenor' of their comments as Judy puts it, to their emotional investment in their own egos, personalities, behaviour and actions. In many ways, the hardest lessons to learn are the ones he taught in this area, to let go of ego. These are lessons in Taoism, rather than in *Taoist Tai Chi™ taijiquan*, though the two areas are closely related as Judy indicates. She says:

> The beginning of the journey was resistance to what the International Taoist Tai Chi Society stood for. One of the people I was reading with some interest was Krishnamurti and a lot of his stuff was about doing it on your own. So when it was suggested that we had to clean the club – I started in a small city in the north of Ontario – I would go around saying, 'We should be paying someone to do this.' I said the same about all the administrative tasks. When one of the Instructors there tried to get me to come to Toronto to meet Mr Moy, I resisted for at least two years. So I didn't meet him until '80 or '81.
>
> So the beginning was resistance and then I moved to Toronto in '83 to go to Graduate School. I didn't go to a lot of other classes because I started going to Mr Moy's classes. They were at night and he didn't usually start teaching 'til midnight. We would be eating at 3 o'clock in the morning so I missed a lot of my classes. Then there was a period when I became very involved in university politics, and stuff like that, so there was a waning there.

Then I found myself walking back into Mr Moy's class and when you did that you were making a statement whether you knew it or not. He said to me that he hadn't seen me for a while and I said, 'No,' and he said, 'What classes are you going to teach?' You see, I had dropped teaching for a while. That was the beginning of my getting it about him, about the integrity of what he was doing, about the fact that whether you could understand it or not there was an enormous, deep enterprise going on, the bottom line of which is to help other people, that this man meant it, he was sincere. I would say that was the beginning of my training.

If you couldn't afford things, or you couldn't go to a class, or you couldn't be at a workshop, he never seemed to mind about that sort of thing. He never reached out. There were a couple of people that he reached out to personally. Other than those couple of people that I know of, it was entirely up to you whether you were going to stay around or not. So by virtue of my walking back into the room that was his class, I was indicating something. I did that quite unconsciously. I didn't even know that I had made the decision to connect to him again. But it was there, and then it started to deepen after that. At no time would I like to suggest that in any way that my relationship with him was anything special. Mr Moy didn't form personal attachments.

He had me do a raffle. I have a typical WASP [White Anglo-Saxon Protestant] attitude toward asking people for money. *Had.* I did it really badly. I expected that if you sent a letter with a bunch of tickets to a club they would do something about it. They didn't, so I was simply annoyed with people who didn't do what they were supposed to be doing. I didn't follow up, didn't make phone calls, and didn't make sure there was a person there who would take responsibility, and all sorts of things. So he pulled me over one day and said that I'd done a rotten job. I flared a little bit and I said that if Mr Moy wanted someone else, I would be happy to step aside. Everybody there went silent and he ignored it because he could understand what you were saying. He especially understood the emotional tenor of what you were saying. That put me on the road to becoming a little bit conscious about my attitude towards money, doing jobs like that and what detail has to be handled. I started to change in that respect.

About a year later because of him I was able to say to myself, 'Asking for money has nothing to do with me, it has nothing to do with me. It's about asking for a good cause. If people say no, they say no. They're not saying no to you.' That was a tough hill for me, you know, because when people used to say, 'You guys are always asking for money.' I used to collapse under that. But as I started to learn, what I started to do with people who said that endlessly was reply, 'Yes, we are and here's why', and you would enumerate all the reasons why you were asking for money. If you can afford it, that's great, and if you can't, that's fine.

Another pivotal instance for me was upstairs here at Orangeville. You see that most of my examples are about learning to change emotionally, intellectually, spiritually. A hundred and thirty or forty people at a workshop and we'd been doing Tor Yus and Mr Moy asked me to tell everybody what I understood about Tor Yus. So I stood up and went, 'Blah blah blah blah blah' and then he said, 'You can talk about it, but you can't do it.' I started to cry and I cried all day – there used to be dorms at Orangeville that were old funky dorms – I would go into the dorm and I would get myself together. I would try to come out and as soon as I came out I started to cry again. The interesting thing about that experience was I was not sad about crying. I just couldn't stop. As the day went on I felt softer and softer and softer as if this armour had been peeled away.

When I went to Mr Moy I was still pretty teary. I went and thanked him. Again I wasn't really conscious at the time of what I was thanking him for, but I knew it was really, really sincere. He tried to coax me to stay for dinner, but I knew I had to go and cry some more, so I did. That was a pretty important time because of the whole coming to grips with the fact that the intellectual understanding of Tai Chi was irrelevant, and wanting to be the knower and the competitive part of my nature and lots of people's nature and the ego and the arrogance. Some of that I think comes from being trained as a sociologist with the privilege of a certain class location and education and all of that sort of thing. He stripped it away in very interesting moments because you could stand there guarded lots and lots and lots and then you would go like that one day and he would just go wooh. When he did give you a whack it was a great compliment that he would take the time because it took energy from him to pay some attention.

Then there were less spectacular instances of this going every day to his class. He switched from night-time to day because the Fung Loy Kok Institute on D'Arcy Street in Toronto was ready. We went at 7 and worked to 9 or 9.30 depending on what time you had to get to work. That slow, progressive practice starts to get into your body, so you start to get the Tai Chi in a way, although it is interesting to me to watch all of us hang on, no matter whether we do it every day or not, to certain preconceived notions of how it should be done. You still see a lot of us doing that, hanging on to things that are actually blocking us from getting ahead.

Without him now the interesting thing is we have to find out what the next step might be for our practise of Tai Chi, especially for those of us who went to his class. The solid practice can move you ahead. When we were going to his class we waited for him to tell us what the next step was. I don't think he wanted us to do that. For sure, he didn't want us to do that. I had something to learn emotionally; I had something to learn intellectually. I got a great gift on the emotional and intellectual level, which I think adds up to the spiritual at some level. Parallel to that was the practice of Tai Chi and then Lok Hup. For a while I wasn't working and I was going down to see him regularly and he took me through the Lok Hup set, which was another great gift. Those things worked in parallel.

Now that he has gone I look for guidance and instruction to a body of people. And I think that will be our saving grace. The interesting thing about anybody getting set up as a mini-Sifu among us is that suggests that one person has it all. If there was anything that Mr Moy left us it was that when he went to Vancouver, he did this. If you weren't in Vancouver, you didn't get it. They got it there. When he went to Montreal he did this, or when he went to Sydney, or when he went to Fremantle, he did that. People had little pieces of it. So we've had to come together to keep it going. I think what will be true in all instances, in the third and fourth and fifth generations of this practice, is that all of the people who want to devote themselves to it in a serious way are going to have to remember that, by virtue of their intellectual ability, their emotional ability, their physical ability, they're only ever going to be able to get bits of it. And the best is when it all comes together.

There were other instances and lessons too. Mr Moy asked me to go and work for a politician that had helped the Society, but with whose politics I had no sympathy. Mr Moy's allegiance to the Liberal Party was a very interesting lesson. He was an illegal immigrant and he worked loading trucks and stuff like that. Actually he hurt his back doing that. Later on he started declaring his gratitude to the Liberal Party. He had us campaign for some Liberal members and so on. I got pulled along by that because I sort of respected what they had done for Mr Moy, but it was a struggle and there was some things I had to work out, but I understood his gratitude.

The thing that I didn't get was that he expected loyalty from me to him too and it was to be passed on. One day I made a comment about a more left-leaning political candidate. The next day publicly I got a real strip torn off me. 'Did I not understand that, in effect, keep your mouth shut when you're with me?' It was a lesson for me in obedience basically. When I look at it again I think what a compliment he gave. He was saying in a sense, 'I've accepted you as a student, in that acceptance you're supposed to be a little bit more aware of what you're doing in terms of your relationship to me.'

He wasn't necessarily wanting me to change my beliefs, just not to voice them in a way that would appear to contradict him. Of course, as a lefty this is a tough lesson but the key thing I came to understand around my Marxist friends – and I am still a self-described feminist – was that the lens that I might use on IBM about women working in an organization like that, I could not use in the International Taoist Tai Chi Society. It is just not the same thing. You can't use the same kind of structural analysis on that because, when you go to look for the structure of the International Taoist Tai Chi Society, although we're more bureaucratised since Mr Moy died, while he was alive you couldn't find it. It was in little pockets all over the place like hypertext or webs, all those fun metaphors that are being used now.

The second thing he did was to ask if I was free some night and I said, 'Yes.' He said he wanted me to go to a Conservative Fundraiser. Inside I went, 'Oh, God!.' I kept saying. 'Oh, Mr Moy, I think I'm busy. Oh, Mr Moy, I don't really think I can go.' Finally he took $125 in cash out of his pocket and handed it to me to pay for a ticket. So I said, 'Okay'. In fact, I had a grand time at these fundraisers. I eventually ended up going to them with some regularity. I just started watching what goes on. How do you do a room? What sort of things do politicians say to each other? How do they manipulate the life around them?

That was a very interesting lesson because I am clear that Mr Moy's understanding of the pragmatics of being an organization, of being a Society like this, is that we have to have political friends. It just goes without question. When we were challenged by Revenue Canada about our charitable status, that just became so evident. Revenue Canada is supposed to stand-alone, and not be influenced and all these sort of things. He just said, 'Write letters' and the charity lawyers would say, 'No, no, no, don't write letters.' Mr Moy kept saying, 'Write letters. Write letters to your MP, to your MPP [Member of Provincial Parliament]. Get everybody on board.' And he turned out to be right.

So that whole bit about politics and letting it go and not being so tied to it is fascinating to me. It was a really valuable time. By the time I got the money to go to the Conservative Fundraiser, I was getting a kick out of it. I was being challenged on this level. Of course, I could just feel some of my friends recoil in horror at the notion. I'm a teacher. This government has just been hideous for teachers and education, just stealing money from schools and kids like mad and handing it over to wherever else. So it's just really interesting stuff.

There were other things he did too that were really interesting. Teaching Taoist Tai Chi to women and men in ways that acknowledges their different physiology all came from him, especially the women and Taoist Tai Chi workshops. People still say, 'Oh women – how come there isn't one for men?' and all that sort of thing. What can you say? Mr Moy started it, the women's weekends. He started the emphasis on women. One of the reasons was that while he was alive men came to train with him in greater numbers than women did. I think he was trying to redress the imbalance of men trying to teach Tai Chi to women in the way that they do it. There are some men who can teach women quite effectively, but a lot of times it takes a woman's eye, just a women knowing her own body to see something. Mr Moy started the women's weekends with a young woman who had, I think she had Hepatitis or something. She had come to him and he was really helping her quite a bit. He told her to start it and she fell away pretty quickly, then it just got passed on to a couple of us. Then it got to be a weekend here at Orangeville. I went to Colchester a couple of years ago and did a women's weekend there and that sort of thing.

It's to redress the notion that there's one way of teaching, to focus on the differences in physiology, but on any given women's weekend here, for instance, the discussion about women's physiology, such as the differences in pelvis shape, have always been about both. Every poster says that it's for both. All instructors are welcome because it's an important bit. I know that there's a certain awkwardness for some men in talking about menstruation, talking about pregnancy, and talking about menopause and stuff like that, but there really shouldn't be if we are going to help each other. A male instructor who has a predominance of women in the class should be saying, 'What sort of questions do you have about femaleness? I can't answer them from experience, but I can access somebody who might be able to or I can tell you what I have heard said.' Open up the gate and let the questions come. In Colchester this summer I was asked two or three questions that I don't understand why they could not have been handled there, but there's some notion that it's a rarefied knowledge now. Nine times out of ten I say to women who ask me questions, 'Have you seen your doctor? Go and see your doctor'. In fact, Tai Chi is to be in partnership.

I went to Mr Moy once about a student I had in my class who had cancer. Of course, I was worrying excessively about this and I asked him if there is something I could do. He got mad and said, 'I'm not a doctor. Send her to her doctor.' That was clear to me that we weren't depositing in the practice of Taoist Tai Chi some kind of miracle. In fact, he stood as the example of that. He got sick and died. That is the key thing. We are not going to be able to stop some things, but we can have a quality piece.

I remember watching him take one of the medical advisers out to see this man who had cancer and they went regularly and they got covered in the Chinese newspapers. It was a bit of a puzzle to me, and then Mr Moy helped us with this, that it was to help people as they are dying. His last words. He hadn't articulated it yet – he was demonstrating it. I think the doctor he took thought that he was getting some sort of lesson in miracleness, but it didn't happen. He was really high on these visits. Of course, what it was, was Mr Moy recognizing that this man was dying.

Passing out of the world

And then there are the people who knew Mr Moy for longer or shorter periods and who were around, or near him, when he died. I am including one account of this period and his passing in this book as it came up in an interview without any prompting on my part. I am not including it out of any morbid fascination with his death, but because, even dying and dead, he was teaching, he still is teaching and there are still lessons to be learned from him, about living, dying, and death. His death is certainly part of his life story, and not the end of his, or this, story about Taoism, the *Taoist Tai Chi*™ internal arts of health, and the International Taoist Tai Chi Society. Peter Turner has already talked about how Mr Moy said that meditation is preparation for death. He has also talked about how chanting and meditation helped him to be more comfortable with the spirit world. Mr Moy's dying helped him with that too. Peter says:

The two week period prior to Master Moy's passing really did something quite profound to me. It allowed me to be comfortable with the spirit world and not be in denial of it or fearful of it, and not to embrace it either, because I appreciated the discipline, the ritual and the understanding to be open to it that the chanters from Fung See Goon had. I also appreciated some of the aspects of preparing for death. For example, in the Fung Loy Kok tradition some chants were done for now. The lead chanter was saying that you want to get to grips with these, as these are really more effective in sending these spirits on the way to health. If you practice the ritual or the chant you will draw these energies in from the spirits and everything else.

I got a glimpse quite early on of this fine line between practising and dabbling in the practice stage, and actually doing the ceremonies properly, intercessions in that area. We have the translation of the last words of Master Moy, 'comfort while they are dying or after death.' The Chinese is a little more simple. The idea often gets modified to comfort those who are dying or near to death, rather than 'comfort death,' including people who are dead and looking after the spiritual side of that. So I didn't know, before that time I hadn't wanted to go there. There was a tough call about that element, this area of the teachings, as I wasn't very comfortable with it.

I remember at that time that I was asked to go down and spend some time with Master Moy in hospital because some of the guys from D'Arcy were spending a lot of time there. So I was fortunate enough in the last two or three days to be in there, to see the comings and goings of various people with experience in the Society and to see what other training was being completed, to be a kind of fly on the wall there, to sit in a corner and watch. Master Moy gave his energy without reserve. He served tea and hosted a room full of people and generally continued to show us how to transit out of the world. He was so at peace in himself and so continuing to make other people more comfortable, helping people who were used to being with him all the time, or very frequently in this area, come to terms with his passing.

This whole area of long term caring and passing out of the world, first of all doing the meditation and centring, being comfortable with where you are at and staying relaxed that we will all die, but more than that, not becoming introverted or bothered about your own health or illness, but at ease with your passing and helping other people become comfortable with that. That whole period was just remarkable, going from being fearful of it to being comfortable with it and having a practical expression of how to help people do it. This is from a person whose oxygen level for the last two years, physiologically, was about 25% of the norm, which I can relate to from climbing and is like being in the death zone, the top two thousand feet of Everest. Everything I had seen him do around the world at that stage was being done on an oxygen level that most people can't even live or function at. Just as an example.

Of course, being in there and getting a sense of the enormous physiological changes in his body, massaging his legs, realising the bone density is seriously dense. The body may be in a weak condition, but this body has been transformed, not just in its total shape and geography and everything, but the density was just incredible. But the subtleties of things.

People would come in with things that had been a challenge to them for a long period. Some of these things were very personal and important to me in this context. On the morning Master Moy passed away he said his body was now open in the place he had been troubled with for years, and he had been working really hard on this for a long time. I don't want to sound melodramatic – just a personal experience that was really quite intense that I haven't shared. There would be a time perhaps to share how formative this was in my own perception of the depth of this teaching and what is possible if I have three score and ten, whatever I have. A very rich sense of the depth and breadth of what is available doing the Tai Chi itself, preparing the body for death – Spiritual Physiology 101. These are just the early stages that it has got me to, and certainly much more important is the way we work together and how we manage the energy in a program. I was much more interested in the Confucian tradition that we have and how that underpins the value system and expresses itself simply in what we do, trying to pick up on the richness of the propriety. Very challenging.

I had a perception of what respect was, from a Western view. I have a whole range of anecdotes on this, but one of the most significant for me was that I was still that way in the hospital. So I felt I could not be just a friend to Master Moy. On the last night the doctor wanted him to take medication so that he would come out of it after the weekend, but he started calling people in, because he said that he was not going to last the night. I felt quite uncomfortable there, because here was a gathering of seniors, his friends. Master Moy wanted to look one of the medical advisers in the eyes when he gave him the responsibility for the long-term care project. There was that level of commitment in the things that were going on, people grieving for the loss of a father figure as well as teacher. I wanted to be there, to watch the whole thing, people came up from D'Arcy. The doctor was asking them to go, just saying come and see him tomorrow, and I knew that tomorrow he wasn't going to be there. I haven't talked about this before; it hasn't been appropriate. Many of these moments were critical to my understanding. These are all formative moments.

Now that he has gone that process of understanding is carried on solely through the International Taoist Tai Chi Society, the body of people that Judy Millen and others look to for instruction, leadership and guidance, and which she sees as 'our saving grace'. The Society is the context, culture and community where health recovery takes place, where the *Taoist Tai Chi*™ internal arts of health are practised and the health benefits from doing so are nurtured. The Society is the topic of the next chapter. Before that, though, James Matthews gives his testimonial to these arts, appropriately in the form of a letter to Master Moy. His story is another of the major inspirations for researching and writing this book.

James Matthews

A Letter from the heart to Master Moy

Dear Master Moy,

It is my wish that I convey on paper the deep and profound benefits I have received and continue to enjoy through your wonderful gift of the Taoist Internal Arts. It is sad sometimes to know personally of people suffering yet somehow they seem closed to the enormous capacity for healing accessible through practice, or finding it difficult to stretch just a little further in their own training. I hope that my introduction to Master Moy and to the Taoist Arts will in some way contribute to Master Moy's vision of compassion and will encourage others to begin practising Tai Chi and perhaps to those already practising to reinspire their motivation to continue to work with the movements.

From as long as I can remember I've always felt very anxious, uptight and weak. I have heard my parents commenting that as an infant and in early childhood I was very quiet and very rarely cried and didn't move around a lot. My earliest memories are of finding the most basic situations extremely fearful and stressful – such as being with other people, playing games, being alone or especially learning any type of skill. This progressed through my school education with me being a poor performer and finding I was becoming tighter and tighter. At age 14 I began suffering from quite severe migraine headaches and a general sense of weakness. Most people thought I was very relaxed, even lazy, because I seemed uninterested in doing anything except lying down or drinking alcohol. Throughout my life I noticed my mind becoming more and more active which was agitated by any work that I had to do or stress that I might have. This made me want to just withdraw altogether.

At age 29 during a routine medical examination for a superannuation scheme, a young doctor recently out of medical school heard something unusual around my heart and referred me to a cardiologist who immediately diagnosed a congenital bicusp aortic valve, which can be explained by likening the valve to a flower with three petals which open and close to let blood in and out of the heart. In my case I only have two flower petals so when my aortic valve opens and closes there is some regurgitation of blood which runs back into the heart causing extra work and a turbulent blood flow. This leaky valve, as it is often called, usually becomes more and more ineffective as through everyday living the hole becomes bigger until eventually so much blood is gushing back into the heart that one would be left gasping for air. Usually, however, through regular monitoring and subsequent surgery the heart valve would be replaced currently with either a pig's valve or an artificial device. This would require life-long medication.

The discovery of the congenital heart condition increased my anxiety and tension to a point where life seemed unbearable. It was like being awake after a frightening dream. I began having quite severe anxiety attacks which included shortness of breath, rapid heart beat and dizziness. This time in my life coincided with some major life changes in terms of my personal relationships and my employment situation. One weekend I was at the house of an acquaintance and by chance I picked up a book on Taoism. I took to it immediately. It was quite amazing. There were many passages that I deeply identified with and had felt all my life to be true although had previously no authority or basis to experiment with them or act on them. Following reading this particular book I decided to look under 'T' for Taoism in the phone book, which, of course, led me to the Taoist Tai Chi Society where my partner Samantha and I took up a beginner's class together. Joe and Anne Chong were our instructors. I loved practising Tai Chi straight away, although I was very poor at remembering the set and so very tight and awkward. I think it was a good show of patience and support from Joe and Anne. As I progressed to the continuing classes and began practising more seriously the Dan Yus and Tor Yus and the set I felt the physical opening up was in some way related to opening up to facing my anxiety. I began to experience quite severe rushes through my body and felt like I'd opened up an internal Pandora's box. I literally thought I would go over the edge and lose it altogether.

In November 1994 when Master Moy visited Fremantle there had been some discussion whilst learning a Lok Hup move in particular that a position of the hands was an outward expression of heart valves. I was so excited by this that in the break I went over to Chris Lewis and began talking to him about my heart condition and the anxious dizzy feelings that I had been experiencing. Master Moy, who was sitting next to Chris, immediately involved himself in the discussion. He asked through Chris a number of questions about my condition. Whether I was seeing a Doctor – what advice I had been given – was my doctor aware that I practiced Tai Chi? In my reply I told Master Moy that my specialist Dr. Keith Woollard was aware of my Tai Chi practice and was very supportive.

Later that evening Master Moy asked me to practice some single whips in front of the group. He explained that the stretching out of the arms and the position of the hands was very beneficial for the heart. He asked me to practice every day. I remember each time I did that move in front of the class he would say 'sit lower, sit lower.' I think it gave me a few clues on really working on that move. Later that evening we all sat around to hear about Master Moy's work with Tai Chi and people with special needs. During this discussion various instructors shared with the group some of their experiences working with Tai Chi and people with disabilities. Gayan encouraged me to share with the group about my heart and what Master Moy had done for me earlier with the single whips. The following morning of the workshop I decided to begin my practice down the end of the Tai Chi centre near the shrine rather than deliberately standing where I thought Master Moy could see me. The previous day's activities had exhausted me, as had the excitement and nerves of being in front of the class and talking directly about my condition which I had previously kept a secret. During the Dan Yus which we were practicing as a class, I remember a light gentle feeling behind me and my rigid bent-over Dan Yus changing. My hips felt like they were sinking into very soft butter, while at the same time my hips were gently swaying from side to side. It was Master Moy behind me of course. It was at this point that I felt a tremendous anxiety feeling and then I just let go. I was no longer holding my own weight or my own person. Master Moy began working on me as only those who have seen with their own eyes can imagine. I was aware of Master Moy working and manipulating my hips, lower back and spine and my chest. As the class changed into Tor Yus I was aware I was doing them too. When I stepped forward Master Moy put his foot down on one of mine and held me in that stretched forward position. I was aware of what sounded like tremendous blows to my hips, spine and chest, yet felt no pain whatsoever as I continued doing Tor Yus. Master Moy stood in front of me and gently held my finger tips. This was enough for me to stretch so far forward. Previously my back had felt like one solid block yet now it seemed to be so open and stretchy. My breathing capacity seemed enormous.

Next the class began doing the Tai Chi set. Master Moy was moving me in positions I'd never been in and common sense tells me I could not have possibly achieved without his help. I remember at one point he whispered 'Fair Lady' and the next thing I felt as though in a revolving door and my spine spiraled around with no help from me. At the end of the set Master Moy invited me to share what had happened with the group, which I did. It's a year later now and once again Master Moy has been in Western Australia conducting Taoist Arts workshops. It's true to say it has taken me a year to just begin to understand what happened through Master Moy's work on me. Various people present during that workshop a year ago have recounted their observations and interpretations of what it appeared like to them. One in particular that has stayed with me comes from Bob Morey who has been practising Tai Chi for three or four years and, as most West Australian members are well aware, is tragically unwell. Bob said following Master Moy's work on my body during the Dan Yus and Tor Yus and his manipulative work and adjustments it appeared he touched the energy centre on his head and torso and turned his hands towards me almost as though he was looking inside me checking his work. This seems true for me in that at one point I distinctly felt Master Moy gazing not at my physical body or even my mind – it felt like he was looking at my energy arrangement – the blue-print of my being.

Driving home that evening I felt like the world had stopped and I was resting on a lovely emptiness. During the coming days I felt so light and invigorated my ability to sit, stretch and turn in my practice was extremely improved. One would have to say miraculously compared to before Master Moy so generously carried out his work. Well, what can I say? Perhaps for me for a moment he parted the clouds and gave me a peek at the sun. He gave me a glimpse of the profundity of the authentic Taoism Master that he is, while to a typically closed eye he might appear to be a plain, simple old Chinese man. I have heard it said that there are so few enlightened Masters left in perhaps these dark modern times. So many people blindly following spiritual crazes and charlatans yet here we are blessed with Master Moy who shares so willingly this ancient wisdom tradition with all of us. More importantly, he shares to the degree that we can be open and willing to accept his gifts and let go. Commercial culture teaches us to get what we can and to look after number one. I feel that perhaps the truth is that as we let go more in a sensible way and be more open in Tai Chi practice and in our everyday lives our health would be greatly improved.

Thank you Mr Moy.

James Matthews, 1995

PS to members

Hi everyone

Well it's probably timely for another instalment of my heart saga. A couple of months ago I went on my annual pilgrimage to Murdoch hospital for a heart check up. Approximately six years ago at the age of 29 I was diagnosed with a bicusp aortic valve. This is a congenital heart condition which manifests as a heart murmur and moderates regurgitation of blood running back into the heart after each beat. The initial prognosis given to me in 1990 was that I would probably need heart surgery within five years to replace the valve and this would require life long medication and monitoring. In September 1993 my partner and I commenced a beginner class of Taoist Tai Chi at the Fremantle branch of the Society. Joe and Ann Chong were our instructors. As mentioned in the letter to Master Moy, I was in poor health when I came to Tai Chi. I felt quite weak and was having dizzy spells, shortness of breathe and was extremely tight in my body. At that time my place of employment had shut down and I was getting divorced. Psychologically I was very stressed, almost to what I felt was over my coping abilities. At the risk of repeating myself I would like to say I was always very pale, uncoordinated, nervous and had limited energy. In grade four a nurse at school interviewed me, asking whether my parents let me eat at home when hungry. I was so under weight and sickly that they thought I must have been denied food, much to the horror of my mother and father. When Mr. Moy Lin-Shin visited Fremantle in November 1994 I was fortunate enough to experience the grace of the master as he spent time manipulating and working on my body. As I write this postscript I am still learning everyday to understand what the experience of meeting Master Moy and being lucky enough to have experienced his touch really means. I don't in any way claim to understand except that before meeting Master Moy and practising Taoist Arts I felt physically and psychologically narrow, small, restricted, claustrophobic, almost like living in a match box. I now feel on all fronts that life is more generous, spacious, open and relaxed. This is a very practical thing, it relates to plenty of air in my lungs, more flexibility in my limbs, less ramble in my head and less preoccupation with myself. Although I am by no means claiming to have overcome everything, I am certainly amazed that almost all of the anxiety and other physical symptoms I can remember have disappeared. It is really extraordinary. I would never have believed it if someone had told me I was going to come through all of that. In fact, just last week a director at work commented that I was completely different to when I started with his organisation in 1993 and was much more relaxed.

Anyway, the year before commencing Taoist Tai Chi following my yearly check up Doctor Keith Woollard (Cardiologist) advised me that the leak in my heart had increased and the heart had also increased in size. He informed me that the heart was under stress. This was not a good sign. He said that surgery was not far away. The following year after practising Taoist Tai Chi and having the touch of the Master the tests showed no further deterioration, in fact one comment made to me at the hospital following the examination was 'well if you're not experiencing any symptoms, then just come back next year.' At this year's check up, following an ECG and Dr. Woollard listening to my heart, he turned to me and said 'It's changed'. 'What do you mean it's changed? Good or bad?' I asked. He said 'Each year it always sounds the same but this year it's changed, yes your chorotic pulse has changed'. I was quite concerned. Dr Woollard said he could not comment further until the usual cardio echo gram had been performed. However, he said it sounded narrower some how. About a week later whilst connected up to a monitoring screen at Murdoch Hospital I was aware that the sound of my heart and circulation when echoed by the machine was far less crazy, chaotic and overall sounded and felt quieter. It was like calm water instead of swirling stormy water. I can't say for sure about the link between my troubled rushing mind and the administration of my circulation and body functions but I do feel a definite connection between a quieter heartbeat, smoother breathing and the speed and activity of my mind. For the first time during this test I had a few big pillows placed under the back of my neck so I could lie on my back and tilt my head right back to allow close monitoring of my chorotic pulse. The technician pushed the hand monitoring piece hard into my neck to get some feedback about this pulse. Somehow I felt so good that I couldn't relate to anything being wrong. A short time after the test at Fremantle Family Medical Clinic, I waited nervously for my GP to read out the report. He read six sweet words *'no apparent deteroration since last study'*. I was obviously very pleased and relieved to hear these words.

It was very interesting to hear Ross Anderson on return from Canada talking about understanding helping others. He said helping others is inseparable from helping yourself. You can't be horrible and mean to yourself and neglect your own health and at the same time be compassionate to others and help others with their health needs. This feels so correct for me. I feel like I have been wearing a very tight suit all of my life and the Taoist Arts are like letting it out stitch by stitch so that there is more room, more comfort, more space and more time to make friends with myself. For years I couldn't stand to be confronted alone with myself, yet little by little, stitch by stitch I can stop wrestling and struggling with myself. As this begins to happen I notice I have more space for others. When I look back over the past three years I can easily see and experience how much my health has improved and how much more I enjoy life. I certainly do not make any claim to achieving or reaching any superior or heavenly or physiological states. Simply that through Master Moy Lin-Shin, the Taoist Arts and all of the people who I have met and been helped by at Taoist Tai Chi, life is not so bad after all. Finally it is necessary to say my health and well-being has truly benefited by all of the Taoist Arts currently available, Lok Hup, meditation, chanting, assisting to maintain the Taoist shrine at Fremantle, Tai Chi, instructing and administrative involvement. I feel Master Moy offers a complete and unique opportunity for health and spiritual training, and the very rare opportunity of direct transmission of these arts from a bona-fide wisdom master. Before practising Tai Chi yourself it is easy to watch others doing it and think there is nothing in it except waving your arms about, but then you begin to practise and become surprised at the positive effect on your health. I feel the other Taoist Arts like meditation and chanting are just like Tai Chi, you need to give them a go. Could it be that like, Taoist Tai Chi, the other arts contain a myriad of possibilities?

James Matthews, 1996

NINE

The Society

THE INTERNATIONAL Taoist Tai Chi Society is a truly remarkable organization. Run largely by volunteers, it is currently active in 28 countries around the world and is reputedly the largest not-for-profit Taoist and *taijiquan* organization in the world. When Master Moy developed *Taoist Tai Chi™ taijiquan*, he did not just teach *taijiquan* – he also founded the International Taoist Tai Chi Society. He created a body of people in which this and other arts, as well as Taoism, are nurtured, taught and learnt. This chapter explores the Society as a community of Taoist bio-spiritual cultivation and practice. Previously, and primarily, Taoism was a monastic tradition. Mr Moy helped to bring this ancient sacred tradition into the modern secular world. The *Taoist Tai Chi™* internal arts of health are taught within the context of the Society, and their practitioners are first and foremost members of the Society. Their allegiance and affiliation are to a Master and a Society, rather than to a 'style' of *taijiquan* or to a *taijiquan* 'club.' In addition to local branches, Master Moy founded the International Taoist Tai Chi Society Health Recovery Centre at Orangeville outside of Toronto. As the name suggests, this Centre is a focus for the *Taoist Tai Chi™* internal arts of health and for the Society around the world. As David Kroh says, 'Orangeville is it.' It is a kind of Mecca to which many members of the Society around the world travel, or aspire to travel.

The Society has four aims and objectives. Besides focussing on making *Taoist Tai Chi™ taijiquan* available to all, and promoting its health-improving qualities and cultural exchange, the fourth and final aim and objective of the International Taoist Tai Chi Society is to help others as the foundation of *Taoist Tai Chi™ taijiquan* is compassion: our underlying charitable orientation is in keeping with the Taoist virtues of selflessness and service to others. Our inspiration is the example set by our founder, Master Moy Lin-Shin, who dedicated his life to helping others without seeking personal gain. For this reason all our instructors are volunteers, and all our branches operate on a non-profit basis. We also perform other services within the community, and assist other charities.

The virtue of compassion underpins the teaching of the *Taoist Tai Chi™* internal arts of health and the other activities of the Society. The voluntary nature of the Society and the dedication of instructors are topics that came up time and again in the interviews. Everyone has a place to fill, a role to play, and a contribution to make; everyone is valued for what they can and do give.

My second home

Genevieve Kierans, who has ALS (or Lou Gehrig's syndrome), describes the Centre as 'my second home.' She also values being able to contribute to the Society as much as she can, and she is valued for doing so. She says:

> I'm here a third of the year. I'm here one week a month. I think I have found the most serenely happy moments here. I notice people tend to get into the habit of being looked after. I can't hold a pen, but I can fold paper and stuff it in an envelope. Doing that is very important for people who are ill, to be doing something and participating in the group. I think that is part of the specialness. It's important for the forming of the energy for them to be actively involved. It's more than just the exercises. It's the spirit as well.

Everyone Contributing

The energy of collective endeavour is important to many members of the Society. Many health recovery storytellers comment that the energy of the group is vital for the journey and process of recovering health. Karen Evans said in the first chapter that she started learning *Taoist Tai Chi*™ *taijiquan* partly because she was now taking the longer-term view of keeping fit and staying healthy. Taking the longer-term view of many other things is also for her a common characteristic of members of the International Taoist Tai Chi Society. She says:

> I like the energy of most of the people who are around the Society. When I look at Taoist Tai Chi, it's about being a little bit more internally focussed and a little bit more about taking a longer-term viewpoint in life. It seems to me that people in the Society are happier letting a lot of the things that don't really matter go by the wayside. And little pettinesses just sort of disappear. They can keep in mind that there's a longer viewpoint and that we are on the planet for a longer time, or that the Society and human beings and the teachings are on the planet for a longer time, so we can afford to let people wander and do their own thing, but still have a longer viewpoint of the direction we're going. So I like that. I like the longer-term goals that the Society has and the fact that people are steadily moving towards them and even though people may take 10, 20, 30, 50, 100 years there's a longer-term focus.
>
> I like the way the Society is based on everyone contributing and that feels like a very nice holistic way of doing things. I think there's a bigger sense of community because people practise together and they learn off each other. I think that the more people that can find ways to contribute to a club, the more they'll feel part of it, rather than something they just pay for and therefore get back, and then they'll become more a part of it. They'll have more ownership in it if they're participating. I think that is a good thing.
>
> It seems to me that we've lost a lot of volunteerism in our society as a whole and I see lots of people who live their lives not thinking about where they can contribute, but thinking about how they can take advantage. It's pleasant to see a Society that's moving in the reverse of that trend. Really, because that makes a big difference. As people are busier and busier making money,

it's good to see people giving back in a different way. I think that's one of the reasons I'm so excited about the Long Term Care facility – I think it offers a lot of ways that Society members can contribute, which doesn't mean they have to be an instructor or they have to serve on a committee. They could serve just by caring for somebody else, just feeding a senior. It's a huge thing but it doesn't require a big public responsibility so more people can get involved in it.

I think it's a big part of the Society to remember that all of our members, regardless of their health, are a part of the Society and need to be cared for. And not just family members. I think that in the healthcare system and in society we do a lot that's family-centric – our families are more split up than they used to be – and I think that longer term care of somebody who has a health issue, or is ailing, or is senior can be too much for a family unit, so it's good to have other ways we can reach out to others in the Society for help and assistance. I think that's good. I think that it's important to have a longer-term view because there are people who have been coming to this one week for twenty years and there'll be a year when they can't contribute for some reason. If you have the longer-term view of life, then you're not measuring everything on a 24-hour basis, or 48, or one week. It's a tricky road to walk because there will be some people who do take advantage of that and don't contribute, but then you'll have to decide what to do about that – it's a different issue.

Even sitting around on the couches between sessions and chatting is valuable. I'd talk to different people in the breaks and they would make suggestions on different things that would help. Just to get to know that the world seems smaller when talking to people from around the globe who also practise Taoist Tai Chi, and to think that we have something in common even if we don't necessarily have a common language. And contribute to everybody else. It's a different way of sharing. It's almost as if you were musicians and you got together and made a jazz ensemble. It's definitely a way people can relate without sharing a common language.

It's a social family

For each program, whether it is a Health Recovery Program or a *taijiquan* week, there is a different group of people attending who are quite disparate, yet they all work together. The longer I stayed and the more programs I attended, the quicker and easier it became to start to relate to people because we were all there practising *Taoist Tai Chi™ taijiquan*. We came from many different places and from many different backgrounds, but we have this thing in common that we have come here to do, so that creates a sense of community, of sharing and support. Karen's experience at 'Summer Tai Chi Week' is not unique to her, or to that week. Participants and Assistants at the Health Recovery Programs at the Orangeville Centre mention similar kinds of experiences. Andy Ferenc says:

The atmosphere here is of a home away from home. Here people meet people of like minds, people who enjoy each other for who they are. It really opens up a lot of people's minds and their hearts. By the time they leave here I think a lot of people change their opinions about people and what they are capable of. They may look like they're visibly handicapped or invisibly handicapped, but they may form new opinions of a lot of people's capabilities. You can't always judge a book by its cover as they always say. You have to get in a little bit deeper sometimes.

I'm not a person who gets embarrassed about asking questions and trying to find out how they are, what they do and how did they get this way. I always ask, 'What is it that you are looking for, what is it that you want to do when you're here and how far do you want to go with the Tai Chi?' I don't wait. I've only got 4 or 5 days. You really can't wait for too long before you ask people as to what is it that they're looking for and hoping for. You can look at them and see that they're really working on that. They're really trying to achieve their particular goal for that week. Sometimes they even go above how far they thought they could go. For me, it's becoming a people thing. It's not just the Tai Chi that's most important, but there's more. There is no Tai Chi without the people. People here are of like minds, they want to achieve the same things, they want to improve their health. It's a social family.

Everybody talks about the family, how well they feel, how comfortable people get in a day or so sitting around chitchatting, having lunches and dinners together so they can socialise, pass the food around unlike they normally do at home where everybody always eats separately in different rooms. Here people sit together. It's non-stop laughing from the first thing in the morning to the last thing at night. To me it's always a challenge to try to improve myself every time I come. Every time I come it's difficult for me because I have to start at the beginning because the MS takes away a lot of my energy and strength.

By the time I leave here I'm on top of the world and then as I progress after 2 or 3 weeks I'm starting to lose some of that energy. When I come back I start at the bottom, work up again, a couple more days and I'm back on top of the world again. It's a roller-coaster ride. I really don't like talking about MS because there's more to life than just the MS. It's the progression that I go through to cure whatever it is I may have. I'm starting to realise that it's not something I can do by myself. I have to have others to help me to reach the goals that I need to reach and I know that I can't do it by myself. The instructions I get from the Assistants and the program I go through each week change my body inside and out. At the last Health Recovery Week one Assistant and I did some great snakes together after meditation. I really felt that we were almost like brothers at that particular time. We did a lot of work together. These are the things that will always stick with me. I appreciate all that as well.

I had been a very active person prior to the MS. Even with the MS in the first 4 or 5 years I tried my best to keep active, to keep going, to keep motivated. I have always been a very active person with sports and activities. I used to be a musician at one time, a photographer and I dabbled in theatre, acting a little bit here and there. I've always had that thing with people, but I just never took advantage of it. I never knew what to do with all that. I just thought, what's the big deal? It's just part of what you do to survive from day to day. I never realized what it really meant until the MS. The MS just turned everything around. That's where I'm at. I'm still dealing with my MS. It's a daily grind of course, like anything else. It's a battle up and down but at the moment I think I'm winning.

The funniest thing is that when I'm not winning what usually happens is that my wife looks at me and says, 'You know what? It's time to pack your bags because you're going for a tune-up'. The tune-up is coming up here to Orangeville. Every time I've done that for a week when I go home, she says that it's an incredible difference. She sees it in me all the time so whenever she sees me down and a little bit not quite at my strength and capacity, she says it's time for a tune-up. I know when she's right and usually I pack my bags and come up here.

This is the most that I've come this year. I don't know if it's 8 times so far, or for 8 months, once a month for Health Recovery. I've met a lot of people, a lot of incredible Instructors. Each program, every time I come, even though it always seems the same thing, it's always different. Everything is always different, the foundations are different depending on how I feel, on how the Instructors feel I should tune my body to the foundations, to the Dan Yus, or the Tor Yus or walking. It's always different; it's never the same. It may look the same, but each time I come here there always a little thing.

As soon as I get to where I think it's okay, it's something else, something else is introduced. I am always getting the hang of something else. It's always fresh; it's always new. It's really uplifting. It doesn't seem like a real struggle because it's always new and fresh even though it may be the same thing. I always like to keep a really open mind to each and every person because it's always different. It may look like the same program, but there's always something different in it, some change in it. I try to keep that open so that I can see and catch that change because that always helps my body to get just a little bit better. That's the way it is. I just love it. I can't even stop laughing, I can't stop smiling.

But come Thursday it's time to go home and I'm back into my business mode. I'm back into the more serious person. I know I'm going to go back and there's going to be problems, there's going to be this, there's going to be phone calls. This stays here. I take some of it with me, but I change myself into another person. I'm not too pleased about it. Hopefully I decided this year is going to be my final year. That's it. I've discussed it with my wife. She was hoping last year would be my last year. I said, 'Susan, just let me do one more year in my business and then I'll sell it if there's anything to sell.' She said, 'yes,' and then I'll be able to commit myself more as a volunteer, or as a participant, or I don't know what. I know there's something here. I always get the feeling here a lot that when one door closes, another door opens. That's something I've learned from the Centre as well. There's something about this place, the peace and tranquility. It's a good place. It really is. I recommend it to everybody.

Whatever J can do to help

Focussing on the International Taoist Tai Chi Society and the Orangeville Centre, rather than just on the *Taoist Tai Chi*™ internal arts of health and doing moves, exercises or routines has been important for other people besides Andy. David Kroh says:

Everybody is coming here for that same goal of learning more and helping each other and growing. It's a very interesting thing for me because I believe strongly in helping other people and I have for a long time way before I ever became a part of the Society. I look at society outside of Taoist Tai Chi and I can't understand some of the things that go on in the world. This is the one thing I've found that I can really identify with: helping other people and getting your health back. Helping other people in other volunteer organizations. It's not strictly this closed thing that's only for us and nothing else and no one else. It's helping your fellow man in whatever way you can. It always seems to come back. It's not about getting paid. It's not about more than decency, I guess. Doing something more. It's not just about ourselves, or just about one person. The focus is off us and it's helping others. Relieving suffering is a big thing, especially in today's day and age because there's tons of it in so many different aspects. People being hungry or physically in pain. Whatever I can do to help.

Most people are my teacher

One of the major features of the International Taoist Tai Chi Society is the dedication of Instructors who are all volunteers (as the fourth aim of the Society indicates) and who help their students, not just by teaching them *Taoist Tai Chi™ taijiquan* but also by assisting them in whatever way they can. Rather than any one particular Instructor Bill Robichaud says:

> Most people are my teacher, and the Society. Early on I was pretty much on my own and having to keep things together in Jackonsville because there wasn't anybody else. So anytime anything was going on in the state I'd run down to Miami and Tampa, and Brandon and Tallahassee, every branch we had, I'd go there. It might be a 5 hour drive there another 5 hour drive back to attend a 2 hour class, but that's where you had to go. I had no other place. That was it in Jackonsville.

> It was more than just the Tai Chi that kept me coming back. It seemed that everywhere I went I would have to stay the night sometimes I would call or send a note and say I would like to attend and I would be coming on a certain day or leaving the following day. When I would arrive and walk into the branch some would come up to me immediately and say 'hello' and they knew who I was. I didn't know how they could do that. They didn't have a picture. This was my place now. They made me feel not like an outsider coming in, but it was also my home and introduced me to someone who I would be staying with in their home and they would open up their home to me. They didn't know who I was and yet they were offering all this and making me feel so welcome.

That was part of it too. It's like,'Gee, I'm going to a new place I've never been to before and never met any of a whole bunch of new friends that I never knew I had'.

There's a different group of people here at Orangeville each time, and old friends, too, that I've met over the years that I get excited to see. This is home to me. It's always been that wherever I've gone I've always gone by myself, not knowing anyone when I would arrive, but yet as soon as I was there I was comfortable and I felt at home. Practising Tai Chi is one thing in terms of doing a set of movements, but it was all these other things that were involved with it that really attracted me to continuing on with the Society. It could have been that I could have gone down to Joe's Tai Chi Centre if I just wanted to exercise, but that's not what the Society was all about. It was way beyond that and I would see people who would sacrifice so much.

I couldn't believe it in my first class. The Instructor would drive 6 hours round trip to spend 2 hours with us each week and drive home late at night and not getting in until 1 o'clock in the morning. I'm wondering, 'What's he getting out of this? He can't make money on it.' He was always so generous with his help and with his time. As I started to visit other places, I started seeing other people doing the same types of things. People devoting their time to helping other folks and helping folks not just in good physical condition, but going into places where people really seriously needed some help with health problems who were dealing with older participants in their 70s or 80s and taking their time to do that type of thing and I thought 'Gee, that's a heck of a hobby'. And yet they were doing it cheerfully and willingly and look forward to it and I thought, 'I'm going to find out more about this'.

A wonderful education

Besides becoming an Instructor, taking a leadership role in the Society, such as becoming President, Vice-President, Secretary or Treasurer at the level of a local branch or of a state or a country or a region of the Society or of the International Taoist Tai Chi Society, is an important and integral part of the Taoist training instigated by Master Moy. Instructors are encouraged to take other leadership roles in the Society and help with the day-to-day administrative tasks of the Society. In fact, Instructors are not just instructors of Taoist Tai Chi, but leaders of the International Taoist Tai Chi Society and practitioners of the Taoist virtues of compassion, harmony, piety and helping others. Dee Steverson has been involved in a leadership role in Tallahassee as the branch President. She says:

> It's given me a wonderful education, it's given me a lot of chances to travel and to talk to people at various levels as I go to the different workshops, especially at Orangeville. I love talking to people from all around the world, especially about Tai Chi, because we all have the same problems, even though our backgrounds are totally different, or even if we have to talk through an interpreter. I really enjoy that. And the feeling, the people. I think that's very, very important. There's something different about talking to somebody as opposed to listening to a tape or reading a book. I like the one-on-one. I like meeting different people and getting their opinions and ideas. You can't just get that. Some of the neatest people I ever met have been with the Tai Chi Society.

Real strength in the wisdom of the group

Besides becoming Instructors or office-bearers, other people have taken on paid positions in the Society to assist on a full-time or a part-time with the huge administrative tasks of running the Society, its facilities and programs. One such person is Kelly Ekman who has been working for the Society in a variety of capacities over a number of years. Like Judy Millen who talked about the Society in the previous chapter as 'our saving grace,' Kelly emphasised that 'the real strength is in the wisdom of the group'. She says:

> An opportunity came up to do some part-time work at the club at a regional level for the greater Pacific region. I decided I would take that task on. So I had one foot in one world and one

foot in the Tai Chi Centre. I actually became a part-time employee of the Society and became involved in that level as well. I did tons of Tai Chi in those years because I was at the club every day so I really focused on my health and I did quite a few hours of Tai Chi every single day and it really made a significant difference, a really significant difference on all levels.

It's hard to keep it all in context because there was so much happening, so many changes going on at that time. I was at the Vancouver club for 2 or 3 years before I moved to the Victoria club on Vancouver Island and took on an additional responsibility with the club as an administrator over there. I was a branch manager. I ended up working almost full-time with the Society and I have been involved ever since in that capacity.

The levels of learning are amazing. I've learnt as much through being part of the administration as I have from the physical challenges. They all offer special opportunities. I have always been a person who has managed their own business and I've lived independently on my own since I was fourteen, so most of my adult life was not involved cooperatively working with groups of people. It has always involved managing, being it, being the management. Coming to the Society means playing a very different role from that. You learn how to let go of that, that solitary activity. One of the greatest, most amazing gifts the Society has offered me personally is that chance to learn how to work with other people, the collegiality of it, the decision-making process.

There's a real strength in the wisdom of the group whereas on your own no matter how strong or wise you become with years of experience it is never as much as the strength and wisdom of the group. It also means, of course, giving up a little bit to be a part of that group, but the returns are amazing. For a person who by nature is solitary, for a person who by nature all their life has been used to managing the show, it's a real educational experience and that requires a great deal of attitude-adjustment along the way. It's still an ongoing process as all things are, but it's been an incredibly, incredibly rich experience. I can't imagine having this opportunity anywhere else in the world as I know it, in my other world, where this sort of opportunity wouldn't exist. There's an incredible effort for people to come together and get along regardless of what their backgrounds are, where they come from. There's a real will and desire for compassion and caring which is the foundation of all the things we do. It's in the Tai Chi, it's in interaction with people, it's in how we try to interact, and we're not always successful, and how we try to solve the problems related to our various interactions.

The whole concept of the organization and Mr Moy's whole concept of volunteerism is what creates the environment for this to happen. If we weren't all here as volunteers, instructors or in whatever capacity, the organization wouldn't be what it is. It is the foundation. I know in the early years people would come up and say, 'Well, you teach, but you don't get paid.' And then they'd be all these accusations about the organization, using people to make money. I hadn't thought about it a whole lot and wondered whether people have some point there. But you realize over time the gift of giving, you get so much more in return. It becomes a joy and nobody is taking advantage of anybody and the whole thing is just a big training and no individual is profiting anyway other than we profit through our own personal growth. The concept is brilliant. How you see people grow and change is quite brilliant. Then you see people come and people go – it's not for them, which is fine.

Trip up lots

Then there are other people like Judy Millen who is a National Director of the Society in Canada and a Director of the International Society. Besides acknowledging the pivotal role of Master Moy, she also focuses on his legacy, on the International Taoist Tai Chi Society and on the training it gives people, especially by allowing people to learn from making mistakes. Just as Master Moy corrected her behaviour, and she accepted it and learnt from it, so members of the Society since his passing need to be able to give and accept corrections on their behaviour. These can be harder lessons to learn than taking corrections on one's *taijiquan*, or Dan Yus, or Tor Yus. Judy says:

> We have to give people the opportunity to do things on behalf of the Society. We have to be very careful that the people who are in the positions of responsibility aren't doing all of the work. We also have to be really careful to allow people to make mistakes because, if we don't do that, there's no training. Every single anecdote I have told about Mr Moy is about how I really messed up big time. I learnt every time, but Mr Moy let me make those mistakes. If you have a bunch of people who are care-taking to such an extent that they don't allow mistakes to be made, then that's not a good thing.
>
> I think there's a difference between somebody who has an arrogant attitude towards their position in the Society and somebody who trips. They're two very different things. If somebody trips and can be corrected or redirected, that's different. I kept saying this to people in the Society because I had felt that we had kind of let ourselves down by not addressing certain problems early enough and I said, 'Look guys, if I have bad breath and you allow me to go around breathing on people, you're not my friend. You've got to let me know'. I think that's the key. That I am going to have bad breath is axiomatic. I'm going to have bad breath, but what someone has to do is tell me to take a breath freshener. I don't want to take this metaphor too far.
>
> We're going to trip up lots. The time that I start tripping up because I'm making a power play that I may not be conscious of, or the time that I might trip up because I'm telling everybody I know best and they don't, that's a different kind of trip, that needs some fairly rigorous correction. There are different ways of doing things. One of the interesting ironies that I'm finding as well is working with a woman who is showing extraordinary skills here in Central Region which is probably the biggest in the International Society, the whole Ontario, Manitoba section, is that in the end she and I will be the toughest. We have to talk some of the men into taking a tough position, which I find very interesting.

That part of running this organization saps you of your energy. It's a very lonely kind of position to be in and you need a lot of support, but I would say it's an absolute necessity. We watched Mr Moy do it over and over and over because a lot of these problems did not originate since he died. There were people with huge egos who left while he was around. I remember one guy in particular that Mr Moy had us follow around the city and teach free classes wherever he opened up shop.

Another time a couple in a small town took over the bank account and the lease, and he went over and he had a senior Instructor talk to this group about the history of the International Taoist Tai Chi Society. Then we left, and on the way back he asked me why I had wanted to come along. I replied, 'I wanted to come along because I wanted to know why these things happen so that we could prevent them'. He respond, 'You're never going to prevent this sort of thing. It's always going to happen.' So some of the training was how to deal with these situations.

We've got another situation in a small community in southern Ontario for tomorrow night where someone has got to go and tell this class that their Instructor has not been accredited for years. Why this was allowed to happen is beyond me. The local group should have stopped it years ago. There's an Instructor who hasn't been to a workshop for 4 years.

Attending workshops on a regular basis is a requirement for accreditation to be an Instructor of Taoist Tai Chi, both in the beginning to be accredited and to continue to be re-accredited. Instructors are still learning; learning is a lifelong process. No one is a position where they can't learn more.

You swirl all around this and I say to people, 'That fight you're having in your local or that Instructor that you can't stand, or the this or the that, all these hot spots, if you want to get them all in perspective, go to Health Recovery week! Go to Health Recovery week and see why we're doing what we're doing. Get it together.' I think I'm learning constantly from people who've been doing it for 6 months as well, but right now from people who've been around for a while, in particular the recognition that we stand apart as a Society, that we are not just a martial arts club, we are not just a health club and we are not just a spiritual pursuit, but we are all of those things. There is a uniqueness about the International Taoist Tai Chi Society that I think Instructors need to become aware of so that we can talk about it.

One senior Instructor clearly says that for a few people who are still around and struggling, they cannot transfer their loyalty from Mr Moy to the International Taoist Tai Chi Society. This is not to say that you would not be loyal to Mr Moy, but what people are not able to see is that the Boards now stand in for Mr Moy, that the leadership structure is where you have to put your trust and faith. They're having trouble believing, and that's very interesting to me, because I think it's exactly right that what second generation people understand, they get it right away because they don't know Mr Moy, is that the structures are there. It's an interesting way of putting it that we must have trust in the leadership structures we have. I can remember Mr Moy saying, 'That Board's doing nothing.' He'd complain that 'they're useless' and he'd say they were doing nothing. Of course, they were doing nothing because everyone was waiting for him to tell them what to do.

To find the line between being self-reliant and still being loyal to him and what he wanted for the Society is tough. And those are key points that we have to know – how to make those distinctions, to be able to start educating ourselves. There's the key thing I think. I met somebody in Colchester who didn't seem to know who Mr Moy was, and that's an important piece, but on the other hand I might not be so depressed by that if she also knew about the structure of the UK Taoist Tai Chi Society and how that connects to the International Society, but she didn't, but if she had, that would've been fine because that's where it's at.

Very social people

Besides all these high-minded, serious and important matters, members of the Society have a lot of fun and a great time together. Both aspects are vital for the functioning and survival of the Society. As Micheline Blaquiere says:

> What I like is the social part of the Society. I like it a lot. Very social people. The first time after I went to Continuing Instructor-in-Training [CIT] week I came back to my branch and my teacher asked me, 'How do you like CIT week?' I say I have come home because Tai Chiers like to speak, they like to eat and they like to do Tai Chi. They like to talk and that's the part I like a lot. They are very joyful people because I think they feel well in their bodies. Sometimes we talk about that my Dan Yus or my knees are very bad, but it's part of the social thing. The travelling around, you go to a workshop in Quebec City and you go to a another one in Sherbrooke, good restaurant, good food. A lot of social banquets. I like everything. Talent night, that's fun. Not-so-quiet Cultivation Cabaret, that was fun. I like that part.

CIT week is held annually at the Orangeville Centre. About 300 CITs from around the world usually attend. Micheline goes on to say:

> The part I don't like is that I realise we are not evolving or improving at the same pace. Some of us are slower to get the mental or spiritual part of it. With those people who are just coming for the physical part I don't have problems because I understand. Some of my friends work at very stressful jobs and they are very clever people and they come to Tai Chi because they need that anti-stress exercise. They need it so badly and they don't have time to help. I think those people are very important people because they help with their money, they're bringing the money in. For me there's no problem when you know what they are doing with their job. A mother who has 6 or 7 children, if she does not get involved with the club, I don't mind. But she comes with the money each month, it's her part and her presence at the classes, it's her part, that's enough. That kind is not a problem.
>
> It's the kind who need Tai Chi to valorise themselves. I agree with them, but not too long. I don't like when it's too long. They don't realise that they're not there for themselves, they're also

there for others. Some of them are very slow to learn that. That's what's worrying me, but it's not a lot. In and around Montreal I personally know about 500 Tai Chi persons and I realize 3 of them are duds, so 3 out of 500 is not a very big proportion! They will maybe get there one day. Me, I like for things to move fast. I would like to help them.

I realise here they work a lot for their Tai Chi. When you come here to CIT week you see all those people from all over the world. The leaders still have meetings while they eat. Come on. They are eating and meeting. They're working. That's why I don't like those who are like customers. They don't see that those people are working for free. They come and think that it's, I don't know how you say that. I don't like that very much.

Between the customers who don't stay and commit, and the leaders who do and who are heavily, if not over-, committed, there is a huge range of people, each with their own niche and their own role to play in simply helping others, as Mr Moy did, and as the International Taoist Tai Chi Society aims to do.

TEN

Research

SO FAR in this book by presenting practitioners of the *Taoist Tai Chi*™ internal arts of health and members of the International Taoist Tai Chi Society telling their stories of their experience of learning and teaching *Taoist Tai Chi*™ *taijiquan*, of recovering, or trying to recover, health, through the practice of this and other Taoist arts such as chanting and meditation, of being with, or learning about, or from, Master Moy and of participating in the Society, I have tried to convey the breadth and depth of practising these arts, the effects that they have had on some people, the benefits they bring and the sociality of being a member of the community in which they are practised. This final chapter is a kind of coda or postscript to the preceding ones. If you, the reader, are only interested in *taijiquan*, or the *Taoist Tai Chi*™ internal arts of health, or the International Taoist Tai Chi Society, and not in how this book came to be written, what other research has been done into *taijiquan* and what other research could be done, you may not want to continue reading any further. The kernel of the book is in the preceding chapters. This is just the shell.

This final chapter is included out of academic necessity and intellectual honesty in order to contextualise, and reflect on, this book and the research on which it is based. The chapter has four aims:

1. To locate *Taoist Tai Chi*™ *taijiquan* in the context of previous medical research into *taijiquan*;

2. To outline some possible future directions for further research

into the *Taoist Tai Chi*™ internal arts of health;

3. To reflect on the ethnographic research for this book about Taoism and *taijiquan* and to present some observations made doing fieldwork for this project, including some extracts from the journal I kept occasionally during this period, and;

4. To situate this research in the context of previous work from a 'health consumer's' perspective about, and of, illness narratives and the healing journey.

Previous and further research

The first and second aspects came up in chapter 6 on some of the health recovery aspects of the *Taoist Tai Chi*™ internal arts of health. As that chapter indicates, and given the breadth and depth of knowledge about the body within the Society that it touched upon, further research would develop the cultural exchange between these arts and modern Western medicine. Other members of the Society who have medical and health expertise and who were not interviewed for this book could be interviewed for a subsequent book. These aspects also came up in chapters 2 and 6 when Dee Steverson spoke about her experience of learning and teaching *Taoist Tai Chi*™ *taijiquan*, especially in her Health Recovery Class in Tallahassee, and about the health and medical aspects. Dee also said:

> We're working with the Florida International University in Miami. They have gotten something going with the Health Recovery people in Miami. They are trying to set up a program that they want to implement in all the universities in Florida working with Tai Chi as a balance component. Where are we going to get the instructors to do all this? These classes will be aimed at seniors. They would be aimed at bringing seniors in to teach them, but also to have people go out into the community. Right now the university is trying to get a grant for a workshop that is tied in with a government agency. I was approached several years ago to become a member of what they call the 'FLIPS' steering committee. At that time that committee was being run by the Department of

Health. It has been transferred over to the Department of Health Affairs. 'FLIPS' stands for 'Florida injury prevention for seniors.' One of the components of that is balance and they decided that Tai Chi would be the best exercise to help with balance.

For this Convention, for which they are trying to get money through the Florida International University, the keynote speaker they want to get is Steve Wolf from Atlanta, Georgia who conducted medical studies that have looked at Tai Chi and balance for seniors. They want us to have a little room to the side practising Taoist Tai Chi. The chairperson has given Professor Steve Wolf one of our brochures. So this is how you make connections, but you need more teachers. But it's exciting at the same time.

I think medical science really has got a lot of research to do with the other components besides balance. Several years ago Tai Chi was used for the control group for a research project and they were surprised at the outcome. Unless you do Tai Chi, especially Taoist Tai Chi, and understand the benefits of it, you don't know how to do the research. I don't know if Steven Wolf has ever done Tai Chi, because he has a Tai Chi master teach the classes. I don't know if he has ever taken the time from his busy schedule to actually do Tai Chi. It would be interesting to find out.

In '95 and '96 there was a lady in town who worked for the Pepper Foundation and she had them fund a research study on how Tai Chi would help seniors prevent falls through leg-strength. She took a group of seniors and measured the leg-strength of the four major groups. We had a pilot program in '95 and an actual study in '96. I became the Instructor. We had 25 students doing different classes that met 3 times a week and we got very good results from that study.

In chapter 6 on some of the health recovery aspects of the *Taoist Tai Chi*™ internal arts of health Dee mentioned her interest in massage therapy. She has read *Anatomy trains* by Tom Myers *(2001)* and she said 'it has opened up all kinds of ideas'. It not only opens up all kinds of ideas for understanding these arts, but also opens up all kinds of possibilities for future research into how these arts access and exercise the anatomy trains that Myers describes. He does not mention *taijiquan* at all, but these arts work precisely on the anatomy trains as they correctly re-align the body and use and distribute force in a balanced manner along the anatomy train lines. Dee's and Bill Robichaud's emphasis on alignment and Bill's statement that these arts are 'biomechanically correct for the human body' have a strong resonance with Myers' 'anatomy trains.' Further research is needed by qualified researchers to explore this relationship more in order both to articulate these arts in the terms of the anatomy trains vocabulary and to instantiate the practice of anatomy trains in them. A mutually beneficial, cross-cultural dialogue about the culture of the body could be set up with massage theory and therapy, as there has been with modern Western medicine. Again, as with modern Western medicine, this would not be for its own sake, but to provide better health care for all and to promote better health.

Further research is needed in other areas too. It could consider the relationship between the fairly narrow context of the health recovery stories presented in this book and the wider social and cultural context in which these stories have been told and to which they occasionally refer. This book has presented those stories located largely within the context of the culture and community of the Taoist Tai Chi™ internal arts of health and the International Taoist Tai Chi Society. A few of these stories have also touched on, and looked at, the relationship between these arts, the Society and the broader context of:

- The mounting pressure on health-system budgets in an age of declining government spending on social services as a proportion of Gross Domestic Product in relation to increasing population (and an increasingly aging population);
- The search for (and use of) complementary cost-effective therapies and treatments to Western medicine;
- The 'turn to the east' and the transfer of Eastern spiritual and medical practices to the Western world and the resulting cross-cultural dialogue between the two;
- The 'Cultural Transformation' brought about by the 'new social movements' that has taken place in the West since the 1960s and

the consequent development of new practices and perspectives in areas such as health, environment, gender roles, etc.

A further study could look at the *Taoist Tai Chi*™ internal arts of health as a social phenomenon within this context and explore the reasons for its rise and success within it.

Observations about health recovery programs

The third aim of this chapter is to present some reflections on the ethnographic research for this book about Taoism and *taijiquan* and to present some observations made doing, and during, the fieldwork for this book and elaborated later about the Health Recovery Programs in particular and the *Taoist Tai Chi*™ internal arts of health and the Society in general. This book and the research project on which it is based is possibly the first ethnographic study of a group of *taijiquan* practitioners and of non-ethnic-Chinese Taoists. As mentioned in the Introduction, I conducted fieldwork in a semi-familiar place, even an un/common place *(see Pratt, 1986)*. In classic anthropological fashion, I travelled away from home to another place, stayed there for a while, made contact with the locals, lived with them for a while, interviewed informants, made observations and kept a journal. I then returned home to write up the 'data' into this book. Unlike the classic anthropologist, though, I am a member of the same 'tribe.' Hence this study is an ethnography from within (if that is possible as I said in the 'Introduction'). This impossibility does not invalidate its findings, but defines its standpoint, tests its tensions and articulates its limitations.

In a discussion of 'the indigenous ethnographer' (which I could make a claim to being in the sense of being produced by, and belonging to, the place and culture of the Society), Clifford *(1986, p. 9)* argues that 'insiders studying their own cultures offer new angles of vision and depths of understanding. Their accounts are empowered and restricted in unique ways'. This account is empowered because it presents insiders' unique stories told 'from within' and gives outsiders privileged access to knowledge only usually available to insiders. On the other hand, it is restricted because it is not an outsider's unique story 'from without' that produces the knowledge of the dispassionate, sceptical, or even cynical or jaded, outsider unimpressed by the practices and claims of the culture she or he is studying. As an insider, I make no claims to scientific objectivity, if such a position or outcome in ethnography is possible anyway. Ethnography is a human activity and involves interaction and exchange between people, and so entails interpretation and negotiation. I am not the subject of knowledge and power and 'they' (the 'informants,' the 'interviewees') are not my objects of investigation and study.

This study is what Clifford *(1986, pp.14-15)* calls 'a dialogic ethnography' in the sense that it arose out of dialogue between one Taoist Tai Chi'er with other Taoist Tai Chi'ers. It allows them to speak for themselves and produces what he calls 'partial truths'. It is not the monologue of the ethnographer speaking on behalf of others and producing '*the* (definite, singular, monologic and) impartial truth'. It is a dialogue producing incomplete and contingent truths. The subjects of interviewer and interviewee were mutually constituted in and by the common cultural and speech community and context of Taoism and *Taoist Tai Chi*™ *taijiquan*. This study is also a dialogic ethnography in that a reference group from the Society oversaw the research and writing processes and the Society sanctioned the publication of the book. The nature of the research and the writing of the results were shaped in dialogue and are the results of dialogue. It is not customary in ethnographic studies for the informants (considered broadly here) to be so intimately involved in the research process, neither in shaping it nor in sanctioning publication about themselves.

In relation to the ethnographic study of Taoism, Russell Kirkland's *(2004)* recent book on Taoism provides a timely fillip as of all the myriad books of and about Taoism that I have read over the past 30 odd years it is the first that encourages those interested in Taoism to acknowledge the importance, and validity, of 'what Taoists say Taoism is' *(p.8)*, and not just what dead Taoists say Taoism is, but 'living Taoists' as well[1]. The present book presents what some people, some

---

1   I am grateful to Dr Peter Cook for pointing out the pertinence of Kirkland's book.

of whom may not consider themselves to be Taoists, say Taoism, at least Taoism as expressed in the *Taoist Tai Chi*™ internal arts of health and the International Taoist Tai Chi Society, is for them. They are what Kirkland calls a 'Taoist voice' *(p.178)*. Although Kirkland is both a sinologist and 'not a Taoist' and his book 'is written by an outsider' *(p.7)*, he has opened up a space in which the likes of this present book by both a Taoist and an insider, but not a sinologist, can be considered a legitimate contribution to the study and understanding of Taoism, and as the beginning of a more fruitful and ongoing dialogue between Taoists and sinologists about Taoism.

For too long Taoism has been regarded as a dead scriptural or textual tradition and not as a living oral culture of 'biospiritual practice' *(Girardot, Miller and Xiaogan, 2001, pp.xxxix and xlix)* or 'biospiritual cultivation' *(Kirkland, 2004, esp. p.43)* as explored and expressed in the present book. Just as Kirkland sees the classic texts of Taoism arising out of what he calls 'the collective wisdom of the community itself' *(p.58)*, so too does the contemporary practice of Taoism expressed in the *Taoist Tai Chi*™ internal arts of health and the International Taoist Tai Chi Society arise from the same source, as we have seen in previous chapters with its emphasis on what Kelly Ekman sees as 'the real strength in the wisdom of the group'.

Kirkland later notes that 'some scholars... have been doing excellent fieldwork among Taoists of various descriptions in some regions of China. But... Taoist practitioners and communities in other regions have not yet received the same attention' *(p.116)* – until now, as the present book considers Taoist practitioners and the community of the International Taoist Tai Chi Society in other regions such as Europe, North America and Australia. Kirkland concludes his book by suggesting that 'vestiges of nearly every Taoist idea and practice ever attested in China endure in the minds of someone in East Asia today,' and elsewhere, as the present book demonstrates.

Kirkland goes on to argue that 'many such people, of course, continue to self-identify as Taoist, both in China and throughout the diaspora' *(p.210)*. Master Moy was a member of the diaspora, as are many of those he taught, whilst others, such as myself, are not members of the

Chinese diaspora, but self-identify as Taoist. Even for those members of the International Taoist Tai Chi Society who do not self-identify as Taoist, Taoism has had a significant impact on their lives as this book demonstrates. This book is not only possibly the first ethnographic study of a group of Western, or non-ethnic-Chinese, Taoists but almost certainly the first ethnographic study of a group of practitioners of *Taoist Tai Chi*™ *taijiquan.*

There is no single, homogeneous Taoism deriving from, and adhering to, a classic sacred text as Kirkland argues *(see p.181)*, but a number of different Taoisms of which the International Taoist Tai Chi Society is one. This book is one take on, or interpretation of, that, produced through the ethnographic interview to which both interviewer and interviewee contribute. The interviewees have told their story in previous chapters about their experience of practising *Taoist Tai Chi*™ *taijiquan,* mainly at Health Recovery Programs. It is now the turn of the interviewer to tell his story about attending Health Recovery Programs. Kelly Ekman, the Administrator of the Programs, has talked about the process leading up to the beginning of a program. What happens in the program itself? As I was asked to be a Participant for the first program I attended, I had an insider's point of view. The interviewees have also told their story about the Orangeville Centre. What happens there? I have included below some observations about the atmosphere of the place and how it runs.

I kept a journal on a daily basis for the first 9 days of 'fieldwork' and thereafter spasmodically. I have included below some extracts from the first few days when the impressions were new and fresh. They focus primarily on the first Health Recovery program I attended. I have related this one to subsequent ones. I started writing the journal the first day after I arrived at the Orangeville Centre. I arrived late at night after 23 hours on 4 different planes and 30 hours since I left Perth. By the time I got there, my biological clock was completely out of whack. I got up early the next morning, did some *taijiquan* and started writing. The morning was misty and foggy after some rain earlier during the night. I had seen some photos of the Centre and the property, but they could not convey how all the buildings and the other components, such as the columbarium (see frontispiece), the statue of Guan Yin and the pond (see cover photo), all fitted together. Looking at photos of them is not the same as being there and seeing them.

After jotting down these initial impressions I noted that this place is a kind of Mecca for pilgrims of *Taoist Tai Chi*™ *taijiquan*. It has a unique history that no other Society site in the world can match. On the wall of the practice hall an aging framed chart of the moves for the complete Lok Hup 'set' in handwritten calligraphy in both Chinese and English and three black and white photos of Mr Moy performing moves from the *taijiquan* set, none of which I had seen before, give the place a sense of home, the home, or a home of these arts and a feeling of the centre, and the source, or being close to it. This was both a familiar and unfamiliar place. Being there felt like coming home.

Over lunch I met with Kelly Ekman, the Administrator of the Centre and of the Health Recovery Program, and Peter Turner, the lead Instructor for the upcoming Health Recovery Program. They suggested that I attend this program as a Participant in order to become acclimatised to how the program works and to see it from a Participant's point of view, rather than from an Assistant's. Many first time Instructors at a Health Recovery Program do this, so there was no false pretence about it. We also discussed the confidentiality of people's medical conditions in an oral setting, with people living together for five days, and the need to respect sensitivity about what to say to whom about whom. Kelly went on to describe the process by which Participants come to the program and how she and the lead Instructor structure the smaller groups of Participants and Assistants. I interviewed her later about this process and she has described it in chapter 5.

I rested in the afternoon and caught up on some sleep. After dinner I met with Kelly again, and she stressed the importance of collegiality in the research I was aiming to do. Collegiality in decision-making within the International Taoist Tai Chi Society is an integral part of its operations. Collegiality in research was a new concept for me as I had been a solitary scholar and researcher by and large throughout my undergraduate, graduate and postgraduate studies. Collegiality, however, had been an integral part of the process designing the research project with the reference group. It was also an integral part of carrying it out in the interviewing process, and even before that in making contact and inviting participation. Finally, it was part of the process of writing, and redrafting, this book.

Later that evening all of the Assistants and Participants met seated in an almost complete circle. Peter and Kelly stood in an opening to the circle. The exact number of chairs was put out for the Assistants and Participants and a space was left for a few people in wheelchairs or with walking frames. Everyone introduced themselves after introductory comments by Peter and Kelly about the program, including the shape of the day beginning with chanting. Everyone said who they were, where they were from, whether they were Assistants or Participants and whether this was their first time at a Health Recovery Program. On this basis, Peter and Kelly tweaked the groups to try to avoid 'personality clashes' and to see who would work best with whom. This process went on for a few days until the groups stabilised and gelled.

Chanting was an important part of this programme, as indeed it was for all the Health Recovery programs I attended, as well as 'Summer Tai Chi Week', though only for this first Health Recovery Program was chanting undertaken both first thing in the morning before breakfast and last thing in the afternoon before 'supper' (dinner). Chanting was purely voluntary, but as the afternoon session was held in the practice hall after doing *taijiquan*, everyone was invited to participate and almost everyone did. As the morning session was held in the shrine, this was more voluntary and less well-attended, and mainly by Assistants. They were encouraged to attend these sessions in order to focus and centre for the day ahead.

In the first evening session of chanting Peter described the benefits that it had had for him, especially for relieving pain. Nothing really esoteric or mystical there, just simple pain relief. From his testimonial reproduced earlier in this book it is evident that he has experienced a lot of pain and that he is well-qualified to talk about both the experience of pain and the benefits of chanting. At the first chanting session I felt a lot of benefit too. I could feel it working into some tight spots and the general sense of imbalance I felt from the long plane flight. Kneeling, whether it was on a low stool in the shrine or on a blanket or cushion in the practice hall, helps to align the spine and it allows the diaphragm to relax, though the pressure on the knees can be fairly intense for some people. The chanting resonates through the body at different rhythms, or with varying frequencies, like a sonar, massaging the organs, and relaxing the muscles and tendons.

After breakfast everyone who is capable does, or is supposed to do, chores. There is a roster of all the different chores that need doing each day such as cleaning 'washrooms' (toilets) and bathrooms, setting tables, serving meals, washing floors, etc. Everyone is supposed to put their name down for one chore. Everyone is also supposed to clean up and wash dishes after the meals. After chores the first session starts with Participants being put into smaller groups, and meeting their lead Assistant instructors, and their Assistants. The Assistant: Participant ratio is about 1: 3 for mobile people whereas in an ordinary *Taoist Tai Chi™ taijiquan* the ratio is much, much higher. The level of individual care and attention is quite amazing. No hiding in the corner here or not being prepared to 'take' a 'correction'. It is this level of openness and interaction that enables rapid progress and development. For the mobility-impaired people the ratio is about 1: 1 and Assistants work one-on-on with Particpants. They are put into a group together and with their Assistants they go into the Health Recovery room that has bars and air-conditioning. Many of these people have MS and heat badly affects them during the Canadian summer.

The rest of the groups work in the practice hall and have their own corner of the hall in which they gather at the beginning of each session. Over the course of the week this becomes a familiar place and the group's own space. The Participants meet their Assistants again and begin again with introductions, saying what they hope to get out of the week. These aims are used later in the week as a means of reflecting on, and assessing, whether the aims have been achieved. All the groups in the practice hall seem to work on the same things, but no one group starts by doing the same thing as another. Despite a range of conditions from stroke or Parkinson's to good health, everyone does the same thing, or does it to the best of their ability, sometimes with modifications for their particular condition or capability, even to the point of not seeming to do *taijiquan* at all.

For example, Matthew, a ten year-old boy, had a frozen shoulder. He did not want to do the *taijiquan* set. He ended up marching up and down the hall and outside in the grounds with one of the Assistants. This occurred after lunch so the Assistants for the group must have discussed what to do with him with Peter over lunch. The aim was to get him to move his frozen shoulder. He thought that he was not practicing *Taoist Tai Chi*™ *taijiquan*. But the fact that he was: a) moving his shoulder with the assistance of an accredited instructor with the Soceity in this art; b) doing it at the Taoist Tai Chi Health Recovery Centre during a Health Recovery Program; and c) improving his functionality in everyday life and recovering his health in that environment, meant that he was practising the *Taoist Tai Chi*™ internal arts of health whether he knew it or not. In fact, he did not know it, as someone, who did not know what he was doing, asked him how he was enjoying practising *Taoist Tai Chi*™ *taijiquan* and he said he wasn't doing any! The exercises, movements and routines are tailored and targeted for individual bodies and capabilities. Although the impression was that everyone was doing the same thing (and in some sense they were – there were no special exercises, or fancy techniques), within that sameness there was a range of different emphases.

The morning session went for three hours. After lunch there was a two-hour break for rest and recuperation then a three-hour session culminating in chanting. After 'supper' (dinner) an open practice session was held at 8pm for everyone, including the volunteers. This was pretty much the timetable for all the programs I attended at the Orangeville Centre, including 'Summer Tai Chi Week' and 'Second Half of Lok Hup'. The morning and afternoon sessions of the first Health Recovery Program I attended in July 2003 concentrated on several of the following: the first 17 moves of the *taijiquan* set; four warm-up exercises; two foundation exercises, the Dan Yu and Tor Yu, done in time together (for up to an hour each, and once a hundred of each in a row, especially for the group I was in as everyone was younger than I was); laps of 'brush knees' from the *taijiquan* set also done in time together; and an occasional complete set as a way of warming up or down.

The ethos is simple and seems to be: the *Taoist Tai Chi*™ internal arts of health are good for you, and good for your health whatever your condition, not just your health condition. This is not blind faith, but is based on a profound level of physiological and anatomical knowledge. For example, the lead Assistant for the group I was in is a traditional Chinese medical practitioner. He told the group that the angle and height at which the hand is held in one of the standing exercises works the muscles and tendons of the arm in a different way.

The week was punctuated by visits to the columbarium to pay our respects to Mr Moy (a regular feature of all programs) and meetings of the groups and between Assistants and Participants individually to reflect on the program. During the second last day the groups met to assess the extent to which the program was meeting the expectations of Participants and achieving the goals we had indicated at the beginning of the program. That evening the leading Assistant Instructors of the groups asked the Participants individually if there were any words we would like to use to describe the aspects we had been working on during the program in order to remind us about them when the Assistants wrote up the individual report cards for us to take home. The following morning, on the last day, we met again to discuss the take home report summary and the daily report card written by the Assistants at the end of each day. This written record makes for clarity and consistency in the corrections and directions given. This level of interaction and feedback is very valuable, but the relationship is quite intense and obviously some people would find it too 'in your face'. Not every Health Recovery Program is like this however. The others that I attended were much more laid back and relaxed, perhaps because of fewer numbers. The larger, first one demanded more organising. The style and mood also depends very much on the lead Instructor. Different approaches are productive and valuable. There is no right way (but lots of wrong ways) to lead these programs that suit different people and their needs (just like the teaching of *Taoist Tai Chi*™ *taijiquan*).

The Health Recovery Program is not just for the chronically or seriously ill, but for all, as we all have lost health to some extent and need to recover it. Health Recovery, whether it is a program or class, refers to a level of individualised care and attention and a high level of expertise from Instructors. It also refers to collegial instruction, mutual support, and friendly guidance from more experienced Instructors and a willingness to work and take 'corrections', accept directions, or advice, on the part of the Participants. Doing brush knees, Dan Yus and Tor Yus together in time promotes an unspoken bond between participants and produces mutual support and benefit in the moves and exercises. Instructors need to be willing to relate to, and work with, people who have serious illness or lack of mobility. For the healthy it can be a scary experience initially to deal with people who are unwell, if they have had no recent or regular contact with them.

Illness narrative to health recovery story

As I mentioned in the introduction, this book and the research project on which it is based arose out of previous work done on illness narratives and on the Taoist body and Taoist ecology *(Frank, 1991, 1994, 1995, 1998; Hawkins, 1999; Kleinman, 1988; Giblett, 2002, 2009).* The fourth and final aim of this chapter is to reflect on that background. Coming out of the testimonials that members of the International Taoist Tai Chi Society publish in its newsletters or tell each other formally or informally, a different style and type of story is being told to the illness narrative that is not a restitution story, nor a chaos story, nor a quest story *(Frank, 1995, 1998),* but a story that encompasses all three or combines elements of all three and yet relates a healing journey *(Matthews, 2003).* These are 'health recovery stories'. The research project collected stories from practitioners about their reasons for doing, the experience of doing, and the effects from practising *Taoist Tai Chi™ taijiquan.* Out of this process a new genre of story has emerged that plots a trajectory of possible, and sometimes actual, health recovery. As we have heard, these stories tell of the benefits (physical, emotional, spiritual, social) gained from the practice of *taijiquan,* from being a member of the International Taoist Tai Chi Society and participating in its activities, practices and programs.

This was a qualitative study that investigated the production of meaning in-depth. The project conducted an ethnographic study of the *Taoist Tai Chi*™ internal arts of health and of the International Taoist Tai Chi Society. It collected the stories of a small number of people who practise these arts and provides a 'bottom-up' perspective, gives a voice to practitioners and allows them to tell their own stories. It undertook research from a health consumer's perspective that promotes and contributes to community health *(Daly and McDonald, 1996, p.xvii; Galbally, 1996, p.183)*.

Galbally is critical of the dominant health paradigm that focuses on transforming bodies to approximate the 'norm,' on postponing death and on changing individual's high-risk behaviours. This focus is of particular concern for those 'health consumers', or more precisely consumers of mainstream health services, who are disabled, chronically ill or aging, as the imperatives of normalising their bodies via health care serve to isolate and disempower them. Galbally suggests that it is in 'health consumers" interests to become independent of, or 'disengaged' from, the mainstream health care system. The new paradigm of research that Galbally proposes to respond to this shift would focus on 'understanding how people survive with reasonable health under very adverse situations' *(p.185)*[2].

This research project has focussed on understanding how people who practise *Taoist Tai Chi*™ *taijiquan*, do so not only merely to survive for shorter or longer periods of time, but also in order to enhance their health and well-being, often still in very adverse situations. It has also focussed on understanding how those people transform their own bodies, or how the *Taoist Tai Chi*™ internal arts of health and the Society transforms their bodies (and minds), not in order to approximate the norm, but to achieve optimum health and well-being for their age, ability, genetic make-up, etc. Individual's behaviours are changed not

---

2　I am grateful to Heath Greville for drawing my attention to this book and to Judith Pugh for pointing out the pertinence of Galbally's argument in her PhD thesis on Hepatitis C and its discursive construction at Edith Cowan University. This account of the argument is largely drawn from Judith's thesis.

merely to minimise harm or risk but to maximise health and well-being. Alternative health practices, such as *Taoist Tai Chi*™ *taijiquan,* are a kind of 'declaration of health independence' from mainstream health services that does not deny their efficacy or complementarity. This project has also focussed in passing, not on postponing death, but on improving quality and length of life, on accepting the inevitability of death without resignation and on practising Mr Moy's last words: 'to comfort people while they are dying, and after death'.

The project provides an insight into the Taoist philosophy and workings of the Society and into the distinctive features of *Taoist Tai Chi*™ *taijiquan.* It has enabled members and practitioners to articulate their experience and share it with others, both members and non-members. The aim of the project was not to collect and publish illness narratives in which participants outline their experience of illness and its medical treatment. I do not have the expertise to conduct the necessary interviews and collect those stories. Such narratives also fell outside the ambit of this project and would need to be the subject of further research. The focus of the current project was on the *Taoist Tai Chi*™ internal arts of health and the International Taoist Tai Chi Society, and on the instantiation of its aims and objectives in the lives and experiences of its members and practitioners. To achieve this end it focused on the practice of these arts and on membership of the Society, on how both of these are experienced. It certainly included participants' accounts of the health benefits they have experienced, but these were not elicited in the context of, and related to, their own individual medical and private health histories. Rather, it plotted a trajectory of possible health recovery in the context of the atmosphere and sociality of Society sites and of the distinctive features of these arts as outlined in publications by the Society. Interviewees were asked to read a 'Disclosure Statement' and sign a consent form prior to the interview. Both of these are reproduced as an appendix to this chapter.

Rather than the illness narrative, the story of the healing journey *(Matthews, 2003)* provided an initially useful and timely exemplar at the beginning of this project from which it soon departed. Matthews is a medical practitioner and lecturer who interviewed eight people, some of whom were his patients or were known to him, all of whom had had chronic or serious illness. He transcribed, edited and then reflected on the interviews and related their experience to his own experience with chronic illness. He is also trained in Ayurvedic medicine and yoga. He asks a number of standard questions such as 'how do you understand the process of healing, given your experience?' 'Are there any particular practices or techniques that you have used in your self-healing?' 'What advice would you give to others who are facing the prospect of a serious, possibly life-threatening illness?' These stories focus very much on the individual, on individual pathology and pathography, and on finding a cure and very little on a supportive community. There is a sense of the heroic sufferer fighting the illness alone, or with a heroic helper, triumphing over it as the subtitle suggests and forging an individual path to health. As with the illness narrative, the body as battlefield is a dominant metaphor.

The health recovery story (the story of recovering health, not necessarily of recovered health) would be differentiated from the healing journey story of trying to find, or finding, a cure. Practitioners of the *Taoist Tai Chi*™ internal arts of health may not experience a cure for a specific condition, but may feel that they are in the process of recovering health. The range of stories that people tell about their condition or status can be placed on a continuum from the illness narrative through the health recovery story to the wellness story. Some people who never have had more than a common cold practise these arts and do so to maintain or improve health and not with a sense of a deficit to make up. Theirs is a wellness story. Others may have had a serious or chronic illness, become well and tell an illness narrative. Others may have a serious or chronic illness or incurable condition and tell a health recovery story. Others may have a mild illness or manageable condition and also tell a health recovery story.

As with Matthews' book, the focus of this project was on interviewees articulating their own experience, including their understanding of the healing process and their journey towards, or achievement of, healing. However, unlike Matthew's book, the focus was not on individual pathology and an individual's pathography, but on the communal nature of the International Taoist Tai Chi Society as the context in which the benefits from practising the Taoist Tai Chi™ internal arts of health and participating in the Society are nurtured. As Jacob Huynh says, it is truly 'a nest for health'.

References:

CLIFFORD, J. (1986). *Introduction: Partial Truths.* In J. Clifford and G. Marcus (eds) *Writing culture: The poetics and politics of ethnography* (pp.1-26). Berkeley: University of California Press.

DALY, J. AND I. MCDONALD (1996). *Introduction: Ethics, responsibility and health research.* In J. Daly (ed.) *Ethical intersections: Health research methods and researcher responsibility* (pp.xiii-xxi). St Leonards, New South Wales: Allen and Unwin.

FRANK, A. (1991). *At the will of the body: Reflections on illness.* Boston: Houghton Mifflin.

FRANK, A. (1994). *Reclaiming an orphan genre: The first-person narrative of illness. Literature and medicine,* 13 (1), 1-21.

FRANK, A. (1995). *The wounded storyteller: Body, illness and ethics.* Chicago: University of Chicago Press.

FRANK, A. (1998). *Just listening: Narrative and deep illness. Families, systems and health,* 16 (3), 197-212.

GALBALLY, R. (1996). *Funding health-promoting research: A consumer perspective.* In J. Daly (ed.) *Ethical intersections: Health research methods and researcher responsibility* (pp.180-187). St Leonards, New South Wales: Allen and Unwin.

GIBLETT, R. (2002). *Fighting disease: The body as battlefield in illness narratives of cancer.* Paper presented at the 4th Cancer Nursing Conference, Perth, Western Australia.

GIBLETT, R. (2009). *The body of nature and culture.* Houndmills: Palgrave Macmillan.

GIRARDOT, N., J. MILLER AND L. XIAOGAN (2001). *Introduction.* In their (eds) *Daoism and ecology: Ways within a cosmic landscape.* Cambridge, Massachusetts: Harvard Divinity School, Center for the Study of

World Religions, pp.xxxvii-lxiv.

HAWKINS, A. (1999). *Reconstructing illness: Studies in pathography.* Second edition. West Lafayette, Indiana: Purdue University Press.

KIRKLAND, R. (2004). *Taoism: The enduring tradition.* New York: Routledge.

KLEINMAN, A. (1988). *The illness narratives: Suffering, healing, and the human condition.* New York: Basic Books.

MATTHEWS, S. (2003). *Journeys in healing: How others have triumphed over disease and disability.* Sydney: Finch.

MYERS, T. (2001). *Anatomy trains: Myofascial meridians for manual and movement therapists.* Edinburgh: Churchill Livingstone.

PRATT, M. (1986). *Fieldwork in common places.* In J. Clifford and G. Marcus (eds) *Writing culture: The poetics and politics of ethnography* (pp.27-50). Berkeley: University of California Press.

APPENDIX ONE
Disclosure statement

I would like to invite you to participate in a research project about the reasons that people take up and continue with the practice of Taoist Tai Chi. I am undertaking this project with the approval of the International Taoist Tai Chi Society and of Edith Cowan University. I am conducting this research whilst I am on study leave from ECU where I am employed as a Senior Lecturer in the School of Communications and Multimedia. I have been an instructor with the Taoist Tai Chi Society of Western Australia for over 20 years.

The purpose of the investigation is to explore the motivation for practising Taoist Tai Chi in a group of members who attend the Health Recovery Centre at Orangeville, Health Recovery classes elsewhere, or ordinary beginning and continuing classes. Royalties from the sale of the book will go to the Health Recovery Centre. The findings of the research will not be used by other parties for commercial promotion and exploitation.

I would like to ask you a series of simple questions: 'Why did you start practising Taoist Tai Chi? Why do you continue practising Taoist Tai Chi? What effect has practising Taoist Tai Chi had on you?' Your participation in this research is purely on a voluntary basis. There are no experiments and no discomfort or risks are involved. If at any time for any reason you wish to discontinue the interview, I will follow your wishes. Not much time will be involved. I envisage a short 30 to 60 minute interview will be sufficient.

The potential benefit for you the individual is the opportunity to tell your story to a broader audience about your experience of practising Taoist Tai Chi. The potential benefit for society will be to give an insight into the philosophy and workings of Taoist Tai Chi and the International Taoist Tai Chi Society. Your current position in the Society will not be prejudiced in any way by your refusal to participate or by any adverse or critical comments that you may make about Taoist Tai Chi. The reporting of any comments, whether adverse or critical or otherwise, will not include your identity without your consent.

I am happy to answer any questions you have concerning the procedures. Any questions concerning this project can be directed to Dr Rod Giblett of School of Communications and Multimedia, Edith Cowan University, 2 Bradford St, Mt Lawley, Western Australia 6050 on +61 8 93706051 or email r.giblett@ecu.edu.au

If you have any concerns about the project or would like to talk to an independent person, you may contact Dr Arshad Omari, Acting Head of School, School of Communications and Multimedia, Edith Cowan University, 2 Bradford St, Mt Lawley, Western Australia 6050 on +61 8 93706459 or email a.omari@ecu.edu.au

Appendix Two
Informed consent

Project Title: Taoist Tai Chi

I _____
(the participant) have read the information above and any questions I have asked have been answered to my satisfaction.

I agree to participate in this activity, realising I may withdraw at any time.

I agree that the research data gathered for this study may be published understanding that I may only be identified with my consent (please indicate whether you do or not give your consent to be identified) and that confidential personal and medical information will not be made public:

☐ Yes ☐ No

I understand that I will be interviewed and the interview will be audio recorded. I also understand that the recording will be erased once the interview is transcribed.

I understand that I will be asked if I can be photographed for possible reproduction in a book arising from the research (please indicate whether you do or not give your consent to be photographed and to have the photograph reproduced):

☐ Yes ☐ No

Participant: _____ Date: _____

Investigator: _____ Date: _____

INDEX
Interviewees